From Out of the
FLAMES

A True Story of Survival

Dave Hammer

Word Alive Press
131 Cordite Road, Winnipeg, MB R3W 1S1
www.wordalivepress.ca

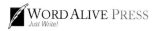

WORD ALIVE PRESS
Just Write!

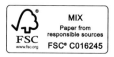

MIX
Paper from
responsible sources
FSC   FSC® C016245
www.fsc.org

Library and Archives Canada Cataloguing in Publication

Hammer, Dave, 1967-

     From out of the flames / Dave Hammer.

ISBN 978-1-77069-337-1

     1. Hammer, Dave, 1967-. 2. Burns and scalds in children--Patients--Biography. 3. Burns and scalds in children--Patients--Family relationships. 4. Burns and scalds--Patients--Biography. 5. Burns and scalds--Patients--Family relationships. 6. Canada, Western--Biography. I. Title

RD96.4.H34 2011   617.1'10083092   C2011-905836-7

FromOutOfTheFlames.com

DEDICATION

To those who feel that life is too hard and that they will never amount to anything, never be good at anything, or never be able to do the things they desire. To you, I say, "Go for it! You can do anything you put your mind to when you follow your heart."

and

In loving memory of Albert Bergman.

CONTENTS

ACKNOWLEDGEMENTS

To Janet Hazlett for all her time, effort, and selfless help in every aspect of this book. To my mom for answering all my endless questions and helping me go over the manuscript time and time again. To my family for their loving support from the beginning of this project. To Christina Crook for her editing help, and Dr. Brian Hodges for checking the manuscript for medical errors. Also a special thanks to Scott & Nicole Rueb, Robin Carey, Debbie & Keir Hammer, Karen Bergman, Cindy Schulz, and Elizabeth Woytuik.

PROLOGUE

The last thing I remember is the girls playing with my hair. It is curled on my forehead and they stroke it gently while I fall asleep.

I wake up suddenly, my body wracked with hot piercing pain. I'm in a car that's hurtling through the night, and all around me is darkness. I'm lying across someone's knees. The pain intensifies and shoots hot, raking talons down my body as I hear hideous screaming. It takes a moment before I realize I'm the one screaming, then I drop back into the deep depths of blackness.

I'm being sped to the hospital, I've been in a serious accident and my life hangs in the balance. I'm being pushed into Emergency on a stretcher.

My brother is with me and the attending physician runs to the scene and takes one look at me before pointing off to a solitary room down the hall. "Get this boy down into that room pronto and wrap him in wet cloths to keep his skin moist, and get an IV in him. There's no hope for him, but we'll do what we can."

I'm immediately whisked down the hall.

The doctor turns to look at my brother. "Put him in isolation. There's a chance we can save this one. I want a watch on him through the night." He looks up at his staff. "Let's go, people. Move!"

My brother is quickly rushed away, and my mom listens to the echoes as the staff rush down the hallways…

Mom has been sitting in a chair since we got here, her face buried in her hands. A friend of the family stands nearby wringing his hands, not sure what to do.

Later Mom walks down to where I'm lying on a hospital bed, which is in an alcove. Peeking in, she sees a nurse attending to my burned and blistered body. She places wet cloths on my skin and checks on me all night, replacing those cloths and attending to the IV that's working to keep me alive through this fragile night.

Mom heads back to the waiting room, to wait until the nurse is finished, and meets a policeman who is entering the room.

"Ma'am?" the policeman says, his hat in his hands, his eyes lowered. This was not how he had imagined this work night unfolding. "I have a few questions for you. I hate to bother you at this time, but I've been sent to get your story on what happened."

Mom sits down, her face moist with tears. "I just can't bear it! If only I hadn't—"

"Don't blame yourself, ma'am." The officer kneels down beside her chair. "Could you tell me what happened tonight?"

Mom can barely speak or breathe; she is drowning in emotion, shaking her head in response. But from somewhere deep within she finds the strength, and with everything she can muster she begins to explain what happened…

THE BEGINNING

CHAPTER 1

SLEEP OVER

These accounts unfolded to the police that night, and also over the following months and years as some of the people in this book were contacted and told their side of the story.

On the May long weekend in 1972, tragedy struck.

From the point of view of Roberta, Dave's mother

It all started when we moved from Edmonton, our home of two years, to the town of St. Albert. We arrived in early May. At least, all of us except my husband, Ellis. We had just separated and I packed up my three kids and we moved.

Kimberly was the oldest at nine years of age, only one month from her tenth birthday. Keir (pronounced like tire, but with a K) was the middle child, aged seven, and

Dave was the youngest at age five. Kimberly made friends quickly with Kathy (Kat), the girl next door, and Beth, another girl from two doors down. Both of them were close to Kimberly in age. Kat had been planning a sleepover in her backyard for the May long weekend, three weeks away.

Kimberly was excited to be invited by her two new friends to this sleepover. Keir and Dave had not been invited, so they were making their own plans.

From the point of view of Dave

A neighbor, Chris, took plenty of enjoyment in constantly telling us that Keir and I were not invited to the sleepover... not that he was invited, either! However, this didn't stop him from telling us every chance he got. He was such a pain that I wanted to hit him. I would have, too, except he was bigger than me and I was far better at wrestling anyway.

I was starting to get fed up with Chris. I was normally a shy, reserved boy, but Chris definitely made me angry enough to pick a fight with him! I just wanted this kid to stop talking about the sleepover.

Finally the night of the sleepover came. This was the Victoria Day long weekend, and there was a fireworks display presented after dusk. That night, thousands would "Oooo" and "Ahhhh" at the brilliant and magical exploding lights in the sky. Smaller fireworks could be bought anywhere for the local population to enjoy, so bright lights also exploded in the night sky from people's backyards.

Keir and I had arranged our own sleepover. We weren't going to be next door in a tent with the girls, but we would be sleeping outside in our own yard in our sleeping bags.

I was so excited! I was going to have my very first outside sleepover.

After many giggles over boyhood jokes, I drifted off to sleep under the stars. I felt safe beside my big brother, even if he did like to pick on me.

I was awakened a short time later. Keir was gently shaking me and talking to me in a low voice. It took me a while to understand what he was trying to say. My mind was trying to fight through the fog from which I had been roused. Finally the words he was saying started to make a little more sense.

"The girls are asking if we want to come and join them in the tent. They say there's lots of room! Come on, let's go ask Mom!"

This was such an exciting night! I really hoped Mom would say yes; it would be so great to sleep in a tent and I was excited to be included with the older kids.

We entered our dark house and felt our way to the stairs. We were not yet familiar enough with the house to find our way around quickly in the dark. However, we found the stairs and scampered up them, then down the short hall to Mom's room. We had to wake her by calling her name and shaking her gently by the shoulder. She hadn't heard us running up the stairs or coming into her room. She was sleeping soundly, lost in her dreams.

When we finally did wake her, she groggily told us we could go ahead before rolling over and going back to sleep.

With a new sense of excitement, we bounded down the stairs and out the door. We gathered our sleeping bags and pillows and threw them over the fence before climbing over after them. We were soon settled comfortably in the tent. It was bright in there from the flashlight that we brought in. I was settled in between Keir on my left and one of the girls on my right.

We talked with the three girls for a bit, then they cautioned us that the pole in the middle of the tent was holding up the top so we needed to be careful not to kick it over during the night. If we did, the tent would fall down on top of us. I made a mental note of where it was in relation to my feet. One of the girls started playing with my hair and I promptly forgot all about it.

I loved being touched by girls, even at the innocent age of five. The touch of her hands on my forehead was heavenly as she swept the hair up. I loved the attention I was getting from the older kids. Then, after taking one last look around, I closed my eyes and went to sleep. I did not know that I would never see two of these girls again.

From the point of view of Scott, the neighbor

I had just crawled into bed when I heard firecrackers go off. The sound echoed because of the taller buildings in the area, so I couldn't quite tell where the sound came from. I thought it came from the front of the house. I figured some kids were just having a good time. It was the long weekend and people were setting off firecrackers all night. I lay down and relaxed. I had stayed up later than usual to make sure everything was fine with my little girl, who was in a tent at the back of our townhouse. Kat had been telling me all day how excited she was about her first outdoor sleepover. They now had three of them in the tent, giggling away as schoolchildren do.

I stayed up late because I was keeping my eye on the backyard, making sure my daughter was safe and sound. I was on the second floor with a window open, and my wife was on the main floor. Kat was growing up so fast, right before my eyes, and being a typical father I tried to keep my eye on her as much as possible!

From the point of view of Bernice, the neighbor

I was lying awake on the main floor, where I usually slept when one of the kids was sleeping in the backyard. My oldest son had just slept outside the night before when we had a terrible storm, so I was a little more anxious with my daughter Kat outside in the tent with her friends.

The window was open in the dining room next to me so that I could hear if any of the kids needed me. The stove light in the kitchen emitted a faint glow. Slowly my eyes closed and I drifted off to sleep.

Suddenly I was awake and wondering what had startled me. I then heard a scream, followed by cries for help from the backyard. I leapt off the couch and grabbed my housecoat. I ran into the dining room and pressed my face against the window. The tent at the back of the yard was on fire! The whole base of the tent was burning and the flames were beginning to climb up the sides. My daughter was in that tent! My heart pounded hard as I sprinted to the back door. By the time I got there, only seconds later, the fire was already on the roof of the tent. I could hear Scott, my husband, pounding down the stairs right behind me as I flew out the door in terror.

GRANDMA

(Writing as my grandma)

CHAPTER 2

THE FIRST TWO DAYS

I was doing dishes at home, in Madison, Wisconsin, when my phone rang. Drying my hands, I walked into the next room to answer it. There was a man on the line.

"I'm calling on behalf of your daughter."

"My daughter…what on earth for?"

The line was full of static, and I strained to hear.

"I'm afraid there's been a tragedy here." The voice on the other end of the line sounded surreal, as if I were in a dream.

A tragedy? I jiggled the phone, thinking I'd heard wrong and hoping to make the line a bit clearer.

"Your two grandsons are in the hospital in critical condition."

"My grandsons? And my granddaughter…?"

There was a bit of a pause and time stood still. It was so long that I thought the line must have been disconnected.

"I'm afraid your granddaughter didn't make it…I'm sorry."

"Who did you say you were?"

"I work at the hospital and offered to call you on behalf of your daughter. She's too devastated right now to talk."

I was speechless, but then it suddenly dawned on me that my daughter needed me, now. "Will you tell her that I'm on my way and will be there as soon as I can?"

"Yes, I'd be glad to."

My granddaughter Kimberly had died in a tragic tent fire. My grandsons, Keir and Dave, were in critical condition. In fact, Dave was not expected to survive, either. I was in shock. The news hit me so hard that my knees buckled and I had to sit down. I was suddenly feeling a little lightheaded.

I arranged to take some time off from the library where I worked. I packed a few things into suitcases, and within twelve hours caught a flight out west.

Landing at the Edmonton airport early in the morning, I took a taxi to a hotel, registered, dropped my bags in my room, and went straight to the Sturgeon General Hospital in St. Albert. I could figure out sleeping arrangements at my daughter's house later.

I entered the hospital with a certain amount of trepidation. I hadn't seen my daughter Roberta for at least a couple years, and she was now in a time of overwhelming grief. She needed me.

Before seeing my daughter, I stopped by the nurse's station to check out the status of my two grandsons. To my relief, Dave was still alive, though not much hope was held out for his survival. Keir was currently in stable but serious condition. I had to lean on the counter to support myself while this news sank in. Everything seemed unreal until I heard it in person. I loved my grandkids. They were such good and fun kids to be around.

When I saw Roberta, she was a mess. Pain and grief gripped her like a boa constrictor gripping its prey, and it was written all over her expression. Her face was contorted in pain, her tear-soaked cheeks told the story of a sleepless night. I knew some of what she was feeling. My granddaughter was dead, and before the day was out I could lose a grandson as well.

I sat down beside her and wrapped my only daughter in my arms. I don't remember what I told her that day except that we were in this together. I would stay until the boys were well again, and that was not up for discussion. Leaning against me, she sobbed the whole time. I spent quite a bit of time with Roberta while we waited to hear how the boys were doing.

I went back to my hotel that night while Roberta stayed at the hospital. She hadn't gone home since Dave and Keir had first been admitted.

The very next day, the boys were moved to a better-equipped and well-staffed hospital: the Royal Alexandra Hospital (Royal Alex), in the neighboring city of Edmonton. Once the boys were settled into their new rooms, Roberta and I went to see them. I braced myself for the worst, but I didn't even come close to preparing myself for what I was about to see.

We saw Dave first in the Intensive Care Unit (ICU). He was huddled in the fetal position on his hospital bed with a tiny white cotton blanket pulled over his body and an IV (intravenous) attached to his leg. Some of his chest was still visible, and what I saw of it chilled my heart. The skin was melted and black on his arms, chest, and head. When he turned over later, I saw that his back was the same.

While we were seeing Dave, the nurses came in to bandage up his entire upper body. The nurses explained that this was to keep the moisture in, otherwise he would dehydrate and all the liquids being pumped into him through the IV would evaporate through his wounds.

All of Dave's upper body areas suffered third-degree burns. Thankfully, the area between his belly button and toes was unburned. I was particularly glad of this, for it meant he would be able to have kids someday. The skin around his eyes was puffy and swollen. His upper lip had melted. Some of it was therefore no longer there, and his mouth could not close. I'd seen enough at this point. I couldn't take any more. The tears streamed down my face as I walked away, my heart throbbing with pain.

It wasn't until we were halfway down the hall that I realized Roberta was hanging on to my arm and trailing along beside me.

After we composed ourselves, we went off in search of Keir's room. Keir had been placed in a private room and he had a nurse with him twenty-four hours a day. The doctors felt he'd be better off this way than if he was in Intensive Care. They wanted someone on-hand in case Keir took a turn for the worse. They didn't know if his throat would swell shut from the smoke he'd inhaled, preventing him from breathing, or if perhaps he'd even go into cardiac arrest. The nurse was constantly moving about, fixing and adjusting cloths, tubes, and other contraptions, doing her best to keep him alive.

Keir was sleeping when we entered his room. The skin on his hands had melted because of the intense heat. Half of his back, his stomach, and the right side of his chest were burned. His right arm was burned, but not his left. Both of his hands and face were also burned, but not severely. He still had his eyelids and eyelashes, but his mouth was in bad shape. Most of his burns were rated as third-degree, with other areas rated as second-degree.

The doctors felt it necessary to put Dave in Intensive Care, because he was in much worse condition than Keir. They put him in a room directly across from the nurse's station in case he needed immediate attention. I discussed this with Roberta.

"Only 30% of Keir's skin surface burned, compared to 60% of Dave's," Roberta explained. "That's why Dave is in much worse shape. Skin surface is measured differently than I thought. The doctor explained that each arm has nine percent of the total body skin, adding up to a total of eighteen percent. The back has eighteen percent, the front eighteen, and the head nine. That adds up to sixty-three percent. But down below his belly button, he wasn't burned so they took off three percent for that area, his lower abdomen.

"The doctors feel confident that Keir will make it and that they'll only have to work on him for a few months. But with Dave, even if he survives the doctors aren't sure how long he'll be in the hospital!"

Then she threw her arms around me. "Oh Mom, I'm so glad you came. I can't take this by myself. I feel all alone in this since Ellis and I are separated. I need someone to lean on and Ellis hasn't been heard from yet. He's still on the side of a mountain and we haven't been able to get in touch with him yet."

Ellis enjoyed the outdoors, and especially the mountains. He was off this weekend backpacking by Jasper National Park and would possibly remain there a day or two longer. The RCMP (Royal Canadian Mounted Police) were trying to get his attention by playing a radio message every couple of hours, hoping that he would be listening and come off the mountain sooner.

I held Roberta close and let her get some of the emotion out of her. She sobbed on my shoulder, clinging tightly to me.

Everyone working at the hospital knew us already and greeted us by name. They had never had a burn victim as bad off as Dave and word spread about him, and then about us, his family. I just knew by the way we were treated that they felt our pain and anguish.

A little while later, I was back in Dave's room. I sat there for a while, just watching him. His breathing was shallow and he lay motionless, covered in bandages. I read stories to him, hoping to comfort him in some way. Since he was so heavily bandaged, one of the only parts of him I could touch were his toes. So I played "This Little Piggy" with his cute, pink toes. I would hold his big toe and say, "This little piggy went to market." Then I would hold the next toe and say, "This little piggy stayed home." I went through all five toes, holding each one in turn.

As I played with his toes, I realized my grandson would not make it unless he started to fight. He needed to fight for every breath and then keep on fighting.

Just then, Dr. Maxwell walked quietly into the ICU. Dave had two main doctors caring for him, the other being Dr. Timmons, a plastic surgeon.

"Hi," Dr. Maxwell said. "You're Dave's grandmother, right?"

It was more like a statement than a question. I simply maintained eye contact, anxiety growing in my heart by the second.

Dr. Maxwell was a pediatric surgeon and the attending physician for both boys. As an American, he had served as a M.A.S.H. surgeon in the Vietnam War, so he had experience with severe trauma.

He cleared his throat. "I had hoped to tell you and Roberta at the same time, but it looks unlikely. I'm sorry to have to tell you this…but Dave is in a coma."

A coma!

"We're not sure what will happen."

He continued to talk, but I didn't hear a word. I could vaguely hear him speaking; all I could hear was the sound of my heartbeat and blood rushing into my ears. Would Dave come out of this coma?

I sang to Dave, and when Roberta came I told her about his coma, letting her know that the doctor would speak to her when he was in again. From the look on her face, I could tell that she wasn't listening after the word "coma." She was probably hearing the same roaring in her ears that I heard, the sound like a wind or waterfall.

At the end of the day, I took Roberta home. She was still dressed in the purple sweater and blue pants she'd hurriedly thrown on the night of the fire. We stopped by my hotel so I could pick up my bags and check out. It was dusk by the time we got to Roberta's home.

During dinner, we decided on a strategy. For the time being, Roberta would visit Keir in the mornings and I would visit Dave. In the afternoons, we would switch. Dave had not regained consciousness yet. However, if there was any chance that he sensed what was happening around him, it would be important for me to be there at the same time every day so he could expect me.

The reality of what was happening hit us afresh after dinner. Roberta kept breaking down and crying, though she tried to do it silently so I wouldn't notice. After our meal, we retired to the living room and sat down on the sofa together.

"I'm sorry," Roberta said softly as she wiped the tears out of her eyes.

I rested my hand on her knee and squeezed gently.

"It's just so hard," she said and started to cry again. "Kimberly is gone, but I feel like she'll come walking back into the room at any time. Ellis may not be back for at least one more day. I'm just so thankful that you're here; I couldn't manage on my own."

I gave her a hug and we sat that way for a while, wrapped in each other's arms.

She looked at me, dried the tears on her cheeks, and said, "The police talked to me today. They're still trying to get hold of Ellis to let him know what happened to the kids…"

*   *   *

Meanwhile there was a crisis at the hospital. Dave's heart had stopped and the heart monitor was emitting a high-pitched squeal. The nurses scrambled around as a doctor entered the room and immediately started performing CPR. Seconds passed while everyone held their breath, all eyes on the monitor. The doctor stood beside the bed, his hands on Dave's chest, rhythmically pressing down as he counted to five then blew a breath of air into the boy's tracheostomy tube. The air went right down into his lungs. He pressed down on Dave's chest in time to his counting. Time seemed to stand still as the doctor continued his work, pressing and counting then blowing, working frantically to save Dave's life…

ROBERTA

(Writing as my mom)

CHAPTER 3

GANGRENE

May 24–July 4

Roberta

The next morning, my mother (Grandma) and I were again on the bus on our way to the hospital, unaware of what had happened during the night. When we arrived, the head nurse approached us.

"Mrs. Hammer, Dr. Maxwell is waiting to speak to you. You can find him in his office."

"What is it about?" I asked her.

"I'm not sure," she said kindly, "but the doctor can let you know."

Then she was gone.

"Roberta, you've turned a bit pale!"

Grandma slipped her arm in mine and we went to find the doctor.

When the doctor saw us enter, he got to his feet and walked toward us. He reached out his hand and held the back of my arm while he led me to a chair. Grandma seated herself and Dr. Maxwell sat down in a chair close to us. When he spoke, his voice was quiet.

"Mrs. Hammer," he said, "we had quite a scare with Dave last night. His throat swelled shut from all the smoke he breathed in the fire. We had to do an emergency operation and put a tracheostomy tube in his throat for breathing purposes. This bypassed the swollen area and allowed him to breathe easily. All this was just too much for his little body. I'm afraid it overloaded his already taxed body and he went into cardiac arrest. Simply put: his heart stopped."

I sat there, stunned. Grandma started to say something, but Dr. Maxwell held up a hand.

"Let me finish," he said. "He's stable now. His body is just dealing with too much all at once and the added strain of the operation was just overwhelming for his heart. We're keeping a steady watch on him. I wanted to be the first to tell you. I must go and do my rounds now."

He rested a hand on each of our shoulders before he went out, and I realized then that Dr. Maxwell was very concerned for the boys and for us. He showed a genuine concern for his patients, and from the little I had seen of him so far he demonstrated warmth for the hospital staff as well.

Once we left Dr. Maxwell's office, we both went to see Dave in Intensive Care. We stood and watched his motionless body for some time. I couldn't believe that this was my son, who had been so full of energy only a few short days before. I stood there a while longer with Grandma, who then left me to go spend some time with Keir. She felt it was important for me to spend some time alone with Dave after coming so close to losing him the night before. I continued to keep watch over Dave, and pondered this youngest son of mine.

I recalled the first night I'd arrived at the hospital with the boys. The doctor had seen right away that Keir had a chance, but not so with Dave. I was having difficulty getting these thoughts out of my head.

He only has a five percent chance of survival. That's what I kept hearing the doctor say about Dave. I also couldn't get the image of the doctor's face out of my mind when he said those words. Even though he said five percent, I read a different message in his face: zero percent.

Dave had always enjoyed taking walks and exploring on his own. When I told him to do something he didn't want to do, he had a unique way of responding to it. There were no tantrums from my little boy. No, one of his favorite things was to squeal with laughter and make a run for the front door. Many times I caught him before he could get out the door, but on the occasions that he managed to escape he'd run down the sidewalk, laughing all the way as I tore after him. That was his favorite game: to see how far down the sidewalk he'd make it before I caught him.

Other times he'd ask me if he could go to the store three blocks away. I didn't like him to go by himself because there was an intersection to cross on the way there. He was only four years old at the time and I wanted to make sure he knew how to cross the street safely before I let him go to the store by himself. I often told him to wait until I finished what I was doing so that we could go together.

Dave had already been to the store numerous times with his older siblings, Kimberly and Keir, so he probably felt he knew how to cross a street. I'd turn around after telling him to wait for me and find him gone. Looking out the front door, I'd see him running madly down the sidewalk to the south towards 121 Avenue. I'd sprint after him and catch him just before he reached the intersection.

That was my boy, just so independent.

I looked up from my thoughts and saw Dave. He looked so fragile and dependent now.

It was hard sitting at the hospital that day, so Grandma and I went home for a lunch break. We came back a couple hours later to spend the rest of the afternoon and evening with the boys. We were taking the bus most of the time now, since it was easier than driving in our current state of mind, and it was less costly than paying for parking at the hospital.

We had just finished breakfast the next morning when the police called. They had finally heard from Ellis, who was on his way home from the mountains. We would see him that afternoon at the hospital.

Grandma met Ellis at the entrance to Intensive Care and led him to where I was sitting by Dave's bed. When he saw Dave, he looked shocked by the sight of his youngest son. His face paled and his hands shook as the realization of Dave's condition sunk in.

In the ICU, it was necessary to wear a hospital gown, facemask, and gloves. Thus arrayed, Ellis sat down and started to talk to Dave: "I just came down off the mountain, son, where I was climbing with some friends of mine. I'm here now. When you're up and about, I'll draw you some pictures of the house you lived in before you came here. I miss seeing you smile and holding you on my shoulders, son. I'll give you another ride on Daddy's shoulders when you are well." As I watched him talk to Dave, I saw tears roll down his cheeks, but he managed to keep his voice level in order to project strength for Dave. Our son was still and silent, giving no indication that he heard. But I knew in my heart that he had.

Over the next few weeks, Ellis asked the doctors and nurses a lot of questions in order to get up to speed and better understand what his sons were going through. His questions included topics such as the operations, dressing changes, blood tests, and all the little things that were being done.

During those first few weeks, my Aunt Mae showed up from the state of Washington to help us out. She couldn't stay long, but the support she lent gave strength to us all. My father rushed up for about a week from Wisconsin. My brother Robin also came. He flew in from Oregon, but he was only able to stay a few days before he had to get back to his family.

The first thing Robin asked when he saw the doctor was whether Dave's eyes or vision had been damaged. Dr. Maxwell assured us that Dave's eyes were undamaged and would be fine. Once he heard this, Robin relaxed and exuded a confidence that Dave would be alright in life if he survived. For a few days, there was a lot of help, but before we knew it Robin and my father had both flown home (my parents no longer lived together). A couple of days later, Aunt Mae also travelled home; she had previous engagements that she could not postpone. Once she was gone, I realized how much Grandma and I had leaned on her strength.

Aunt Mae had served for ten years as a nurse in the army corps with such titles as "Head Nurse of Medical and Surgical Floors" and "Head Nurse of Out-Patient Clinics." Afterwards, she took additional training and specialized in surgical nursing. She served in several army and civilian hospitals in New York, Boston, Denver, and San Francisco. She had seen it all and exuded confidence that the boys would make it. She knew her way around hospital procedures and we'd come to rely on her more than we knew.

Things rapidly got back to normal after all the extra help had gone.

One night shortly after, I was up several times, sick with the flu. By morning, I was in no shape to be going to the hospital. The boys were very susceptible to sickness in their condition, especially Dave, so Grandma went by herself that day. Ellis went in to help her with the boys for the couple days I stayed home. Ellis taught at the college level, therefore classes had already ended. This gave him a flexible schedule to be with the boys when he wasn't in meetings or preparing his fall courses.

Many weeks passed before the doctors were able to stabilize Dave enough to perform surgery. Even though he'd been admitted to the hospital on May 22, the doctors didn't do any work on his burns in surgery until June

8. From that point forward, he was in surgery a lot. Skin was removed from below his waist (the unburned area) and placed onto his upper body. When it wasn't possible for the doctors to use Dave's own skin, they used donor skin that people generously donated from their own body. Dave's body rejected the donor skin, but it did buy time for his own skin to grow back on his lower body so that it could be used again.

Infection then set into the skin of his upper body and the doctors had to do more skin grafts to replace the infected skin. Dave's hands were in extremely bad shape and were completely black from the burns. The doctors were doing their best to save them when they discovered that gangrene had set in. Gangrene is the dying of tissue where blood cells are damaged so badly that they can no longer circulate blood.

This was the case in Dave's fingers, which were burned so badly that the tissue was dead. If not removed (amputated), they would become infected, spread, and eventually result in a much larger area needing amputation. In order to save as much healthy tissue as possible, all his fingers were amputated down to the second knuckle.

I was concerned about this, so I searched for one of the doctors. I found Dr. Maxwell and asked him what he thought Dave's life would be like once he was released from the hospital.

"You have to realize that Dave is not out of danger yet," Dr. Maxwell said. "We are keeping ahead of the infection now, but it will get worse before it gets better." He then explained that burn victims go through four stages. "The first stage is shock; second is acute infection; third, chronic infection; and fourth, muscle contraction. Both boys are in the third stage. Dave is very thin and weak. I don't know how much more his body can take."

"But his hands?" I implored him. "What do you think about his hands?"

"Listen," he said, "I sincerely hope that I'm proved wrong on this, but the way I see it he will always be totally handicapped with his hands. However, we'll do what we can to make his hands as functional as possible."

Then, changing the subject, he added, "I want to tell you that I am very impressed by your faith in regards to Dave. All you can do is nudge him along, encourage him, and think of creative ways for him to do things. Given time, he'll probably come to think of his own ways to do things, and if he is determined and creative enough, he'll surpass many people's expectations."

That night, Grandma and I discussed what the doctor had said. We decided to support Dave in every way possible. Grandma also decided to stay for as long as I needed her, though she hoped it wouldn't be indefinitely. She'd dropped everything to come and did need to get back home at some point.

Because of Grandma's decision to stay, she made the call to resign from the library where she worked in Wisconsin. She didn't know when she would be going home and therefore felt this was the best course of action.

One morning shortly afterward, Grandma and I arrived at the hospital a bit earlier than usual. We both went to check in on Dave. He had gone for an operation earlier, but we figured he would be back in his room by now.

As we headed down the hall, we saw a flurry of activity down near the end. We couldn't tell whose room it was and, curious, kept walking. As we got closer, we realized the nurses were coming in and out of Dave's room. The first thing we noticed when we entered the room were the nurses around Dave's bed, talking to him.

Once we reached the bed we peered past the nurses and saw that Dave's eyes were open. He was awake! We squeezed past them, and in our gowns and gloves gave him tender hugs so as not to hurt him. Then Grandma and I gave each other a hug, and danced around celebrating.

Relief flooded through me like a rushing river. Seeing Dave awake lifted my spirits, but I knew there was still a long way to go before he was out of danger. He was still in critical condition.

He spent many more weeks in the ICU, because he was too susceptible to germs and the doctors feared that if he shared a room he would catch other patients' sicknesses. A simple cold, the doctors were sure, would overload his already taxed body and might even kill him.

CHAPTER 4

. . . .

THE PSYCHOLOGIST

July 4–July 31

Roberta

Dave was out of his coma and growing stronger, but ever so slowly. He had been in the coma for six weeks and his body was extremely weak, so every tiny bit of energy that entered his body increased his chance of survival. He was heavily sedated to minimize his pain. Even though he was no longer in a coma, he was unconscious most of the time. He did have his moments of wakefulness, and during these times he would usually ask for something to eat or drink.

Dave was so skinny at this point that the nurses were determined to fatten him up. The doctors ordered that a gastrostomy tube be inserted through his stomach in order to get more food into his body. At mealtime, the nurses would come in with a bag of liquid food, hang it from a metal stand, and attach this tube to the one in his stomach. As the nurses poured his food through the tube and into his belly, I could see his little tummy starting to swell.

"He's had enough," I would say.

"Just a little bit more," the nurses would chirp while his stomach rose even higher until it was tight, round, and sticking out.

"That's too much!"

The nurses then stopped and Dave promptly threw it all up because his stomach was *too* full. Then the feeding process would start all over again, but this time the nurses would fill his stomach up a little less. They always tried to get as much food in him as possible, to put meat on his frail little body. Similar episodes happened numerous times.

June had been a blur, each day different, no two the same. Dave's breathing tube had been removed. It had originally been inserted because his throat had swollen up from the all the smoke from the fire. Now his throat had returned to normal and the tube was no longer necessary.

The infections were challenging for Dave's body, so although the feeding tube was used, it was only necessary long enough to fatten him up a bit. Once it was removed, we spent our days feeding him and reading to him. We once even brought Dave fresh-baked gingerbread, full of molasses. He loved it! It was wonderful to see his appetite improving.

By July, Dave had gone through four operations on his eyelids alone, but the area was so small that the skin added onto the lid shrank quickly and would not remain.

At the end of the first week of July, seven weeks after the fire, the nurses cranked up Dave's bed so that he could sit up for the first time. It was very exciting to see.

Keir was improving rapidly and began to walk around after spending over a month in the hospital bed. He could get out of bed by himself, walk to the chair, and wait there while the nurse made his bed. He was improving nicely and was just now starting to fill out and put on some weight.

The doctors thought Keir had undergone his last surgery by the end of July. They were aiming for him to be moved to a children's hospital by mid-September, where he could receive physical therapy for a few weeks. He was getting some physical therapy already, but he would be able to get more one-on-one training at the children's hospital. After that, he would be ready to go home. As for Dave, nobody knew yet when he might be going home.

During the moments when Dave was awake and alert, he was under the care of a psychologist to assess if the fire had caused any brain damage. Most importantly, the psychologist wanted to see if there was anything he could do to improve Dave's life. I knew Dave was seeing the psychologist, but I was apprehensive about meeting him myself. I wanted my son to live, but I did not want him to live with mental difficulties because of the horror of the fire. I was therefore scared of what the psychologist might have found during his time with Dave.

One day, the psychologist and I bumped into each other in the hall. He cleared his throat as if he had something to say, but did not speak.

"Is there something you want to ask me, Doctor?" I asked, looking at him and feeling a bit uneasy.

"As you know," he said., "I have been spending some time with your younger son. Both of your sons, actually, but it is the younger one I wish to talk to you about. I don't know any way to do this except to just say it. It is my opinion that it would be far better if your son did not survive. If he survives, he will be a burden to you and totally dependent upon you for the rest of his life. You could be looking at a good fifty to seventy years…"

The devastation I'd been dealing with was more than I could bear. I didn't need this added burden. I felt close to losing control of myself and was barely managing to keep my composure. My eyes welled up with tears and I turned and walked away. I couldn't speak. The emotions raging inside of me were slicing my heart. I was shocked he would even suggest that I just let Dave die.

My little baby boy! It can't happen…it just can't!

It had been a hard road for me, trying to keep my spirits up during this nightmare. What the psychologist shared with me deflated me entirely. I felt small and helpless.

How could he have said such a thing? I just could not bear to think about it.

I went on like this, refusing to take a look at the issue, until one day the bomb went off. And the questions pounded in my skull.

Had it been worth it? Calling up friends and relatives to pray, pray, pray? Spending all my time exhorting him?

"Come on, Dave, you can do it!"

"It will be all right."

"You're going to make it!"

"You're going to be okay!"

"You'll survive."

"Keep fighting!"

"You're coming through."

In fact, Ellis and I had been saying these things to him for months as he lay in bed, first in a coma, then drugged up. Was it true that it had all been in vain? Should I have started to tell him that it was okay to give up and quit? Should I have just given up after all this fighting? These questions raged in my mind.

Even if I gave up fighting for him, I decided that I couldn't tell him that it might be better if he didn't live. No, I would not tell Dave this! Was I going to give up fighting for him, though?

Finally, the questions ceased. The smoke cleared, and I was raging mad. *How dare that psychologist tell me such a thing!*

Dave maybe wouldn't make it, but negative thinking would only create negative effects. This was the time to fight and believe in Dave.

I resolved then and there to keep on encouraging Dave and believe that he would survive and live a life full of fun, excitement, and encouragement, with friendships and love.

In my heart, I looked into the future. I saw my boy running and playing and laughing his melodious laugh that warmed everybody's heart. I saw him sharing how he'd overcome all the obstacles in his life. Fun and excitement shone on his face. I saw him surrounded by friends who raised him up on their shoulders when he couldn't lift himself.

Despite his scars, I saw the sweetest of girls with her arm linked in his, her face turned towards him laughing at one of the witty comments he was always coming up with. Charm and warmth radiated out of her. I saw his life surrounded with laughter and goodness and his heart full with all the good things in life. I saw it all in a lightning flash and I purposed that my sweet little boy was going to have me behind him every step of the way.

It wasn't until much later that I was able to get over the words of the psychologist and get my spirits back up. He had said that Dave would be a burden on us for fifty to seventy years, but as it turned out, Dave was not dependent on us for much longer.

CHAPTER 5

KEIR'S RECOLLECTIONS

August 1–August 31

Roberta

The months passed slowly. Each day held new challenges and heartache. I had no idea how I would have managed without all of Grandma's help with the boys. She visited Keir in the mornings now while I visited Dave and fed him at lunchtime. In the afternoon, Grandma sometimes got a little free time while I visited Keir.

I was not always able to visit Keir, though, especially if Dave needed me or if he was coming back from an operation or debridement session, both of which took place in the operating room. Debridement is the removal of dead, hardened skin from the body and can be so painful that it needs to be done under anesthetic. I often waited for Dave so that I would be there for him when he got back to his room.

Dave invariably asked for a drink as soon as he woke up after surgery. He'd request apple juice or ginger ale, often falling sound asleep before his drink came. When he was awake, the drink didn't often stay down because his stomach was still upset from the anesthetic.

I'd often cry for hours while sitting beside Dave's bed, watching his chest rise and fall. His breathing was barely noticeable in the room, and his body still and horribly marred. It was hard to see him this way, when I remembered him so healthy. I tried to cry silently so as not to wake him, but at night, with only Grandma in the house, I could let myself go; I could let out all the overwhelming emotions of the day.

Dave continued to lie in bed, immobile, a far cry from his usual independent self. His exuberance and delight in life lay buried somewhere deep within him. And on he slept. Sleep seemed to be his way of escaping from the pain and horror. It was more than I could take, seeing him like this, but then everything was more than I could take. However, even though I didn't think I could, I somehow managed to survive each day.

Sitting next to Dave's bed, I recalled the night of the fire. Dave's entire upper body had been completely blackened from the fire. Roy, a neighbor from the house at the corner, had driven us to the hospital. Keir was lying on the back seat of their station wagon. I was beside him with

Dave across my knees. Dave only woke up once during that trip. His skin was melting from the heat of the fire and he screamed from the pain and passed out.

Before the fire, Dave preferred to explore, go for walks by himself, and learn things on his own. Yet here he lay, totally dependent on us.

I spent a lot of time sitting beside Dave's bed, not just watching him, but reading and singing to him in order to let him know I was there. I knew his subconscious mind would catch what I said even if he was asleep or drugged. His mind had nothing with which to occupy itself except dreams, so I engaged his mind by reading to him. He always seemed to rest much better when I spent time with him in this way.

By the end of August, Dave had gone through approximately thirty operations. There seemed to be no end in sight. His condition was still serious and he had a long road ahead of him. He was much more alert when he was awake, though some days he was easily worn out.

The days were long. Oftentimes when Grandma and I got back to the house, we didn't have the energy to talk. But occasionally we had a rather long conversation in the evening.

One particular night, Grandma told me a rather interesting story:

"You know," she said, "Keir told me something rather peculiar today. I'm surprised he hadn't mentioned it earlier... We were talking about Dave, because he's very concerned about him and always wants to know how he's doing. So I was telling him about some of the operations that Dave had just gone through. Suddenly he turned to me, his face all serious, and said, 'Dave was crying in the tent that night, you know. I couldn't see him through the flames, but I could hear him crying.'

"I waited to hear what Keir was going to say next, scarcely daring to breathe because I didn't want to miss a word. Then he continued: 'I wanted to help him, so I reached through the flames with my right arm until I felt him and then grabbed hold of him and pulled him through those flames until he was beside me. And you know what, Grandma? When he was beside me and could see me, he stopped crying.'

"Then the oddest thing happened, Roberta. Keir started crying and uttered these words that took me completely off-guard. 'I miss him,' he said between sobs. 'I want to see him!'"

CHAPTER 6

PNEUMONIA

September 1–October 1

Roberta

I realized that pulling Dave through the flames was probably why Keir's right arm had been burned. By reaching through the flames, Keir had probably saved his little brother's life. It brought tears to my eyes as Grandma relayed the story, because it seemed as though the hand of God had pulled Dave through those flames.

Throughout these emotionally trying months, there was a song playing on the radio that gave me something to cling to. Every time I heard it, peace would wash over me like a refreshing waterfall. The song was "Amazing Grace" and it played over and over again each day. It helped me in this time of feeling untethered, when nothing in life was making any sense. I felt as if I were being swept all over the place in a raging torrent; my mind just could not grasp the full reality of what had happened to my children, and that song helped keep me together. I needed grace in my life each day to keep going.

By early September, Dave had come a long way, but Grandma and I still weren't sure if he had enough strength and determination for the long haul. He was very sickly, thin, and easily tired. One evening, while Grandma and I sat at home resting from the ordeals of the day, she suddenly slapped her knee and blurted out, "When is that boy going to start to fight?"

I looked at her questioningly, wondering which of my two boys she was referring to.

"I'm talking about Dave," she said as if reading my thoughts. "If he doesn't start fighting soon, it may be too late…"

I knew what she meant. I really believed that Dave would make it, but unless he started to fight, there was but a small chance he would even live past the month. None of the doctors had believed he would even make it this far.

Ellis worked out his schedule so that when Grandma and I left for the day, he came in to visit the boys. He did this during the week, and on weekends he often went mountain climbing. He seemed to have a hard time dealing with the tragedy and seeing his sons in that condition, but he came to the hospital more and more frequently, and this helped lighten the load for the rest of us. Although

Dave was awake much more often now that he was taken off all the drugs, he still needed a lot of sleep to help his little body heal. More and more, Dave loved being read to. He had an insatiable appetite for books and was always looking forward to the next one. His favorite book at the time was *The Shoemaker and the Elves*, by the famous Grimm brothers. I read it to him at least twice a day.

One day while I was visiting Keir, he asked, "When can I visit Dave? I want to see how my brother's doing."

"He's in Intensive Care, honey," I said. "No one is allowed to visit him except Grandma, Daddy, and me. Once he's put into a regular room, you'll be able to see him."

"But how is he doing? Will he be okay?" His face was scrunched up with concern and he had tears in his eyes.

I didn't want to worry Keir, but I also didn't want to get his hopes up only to have them dashed, either. "We don't know yet. We'll just have to wait and see." I rested my hand on his. "The doctors are happy with how Dave is doing right now and they hope to move him out of ICU soon and up to the children's ward. As soon as he's up there, you'll be able to visit him."

Occasionally Grandma and I got a day off from the hospital, and it was nice to be somewhere else for that one day. As much as I loved my sons, it was necessary to have a break now and again. One particular week we got two days off, and on the first day we went for a walk in the woods, got lost, and couldn't find our way back to the car. We could see it in the distance though, through the dense brush. We finally ended up crawling through a hole in the fence to get back to the car. It was much-needed fun that we had together that day.

On the second day, we went on a shopping spree and went a little crazy with the sales we found. We came home at the end with five cents left. It was nice for the two of us to spend those days together and just for a moment to forget everything that was happening in the hospital.

The following day, we were back at the hospital. Dave was due for another surgery and it was really at that point that I began to see the little fighter in him. He was fighting through the ordeals and making good progress. I was so proud of him! He was also becoming very talkative, which was encouraging, but only time would tell whether he had the endurance for the long road ahead.

The day finally arrived when Dave was moved up to the children's ward on the second floor. I was thrilled. It showed just how fast he was getting better and stronger before our very eyes. He would still be in isolation, meaning everything going in and out of his room would be sterilized, but at least both boys would be in the same wing of the hospital. The food was much better for Dave in the children's ward, too, as it was made especially for him. This helped keep him well-nourished and healing.

I remember the day well that the nurse set Dave on my lap while she changed the bed. All the moving was quite painful for him, but he must have enjoyed being in my arms, because he asked to sit on my lap again the very next day. It was a mixture of pain and pleasure for me as I held Dave fully in my arms for the first time in months. Tears trickled down my face as I experienced the joy of holding him, yet I felt his pain and anguish as well.

My main hardship was watching Dave and Keir's pain hour by hour. I just wished I could take it all away from them.

Within a short time, the doctors saw that Dave was doing much better than they had expected, so he was moved into a ward with several other children.

One fall day stood out from the rest. Arriving at the hospital, I went to see Dave, but he wasn't there. I went to check at the nurse's station, and that's when I saw him being wheeled back to his room from the bath. His skin was still moist and he was wearing only a thin white hospital gown. The halls were cold and chilly.

"What are you doing?" I asked the nurses, anger filling my voice.

I walked beside them back to Dave's room. I was furious and waited in the hall while they put Dave safely back in bed. When they came out of his room, I let them have it.

"What were you thinking? Don't you realize that he needs to be kept warm at all times? And yet you bring him back from a bath down these cold, breezy halls with nothing more than a thin gown to cover him?"

The nurses were looking ashamed at this point.

"Don't ever do that again!" With that, I stormed off, leaving them speechless.

Once I'd cooled off a bit, I went in to see Dave. I noticed the boy in the next bed had a cold but didn't think too much of it at the time. I should have.

The very next day, Dave caught a cold and within a day or two the cold moved into his lungs and he had full-blown pneumonia. The doctors and nurses were extremely upset with themselves over this. After all their hard work and countless hours getting him well, in one moment they'd nullified everything by moving him into a room too soon with other children. All of Dave's progress was pushed right back to square one.

Dave was promptly relocated in an isolated room and placed in an oxygen tent. I looked at him in that tent, his frail body shivering against the cold air being pumped inside, a thin blanket clutched in his hands that barely covered his frail body.

The tent was essentially a clear plastic sheet suspended over the bed, then tucked beneath the mattress to make a tight seal. Streams of chilly air were blown into Dave's world inside this structure. Zippers on the sides of it gave the nurses access to him. It was similar to a cold air humidifier, giving him plenty of moist air to help his breathing.

I stood in the doorway as everything was being set up and leaned against the door jamb. My mind reeled. He had been making such progress. How could this happen now?

The doctor suddenly steered me to a place where he could talk to me privately.

"We don't think your boy is going to make it," he said. "It's very unlikely that his body will withstand this in his current condition. Another couple of months and he might have. At this point, we'd be very surprised."

Having already lost my daughter Kimberly, I was terrified of losing another child. I didn't think my heart could take it.

Each day, Dave huddled in his little blanket and shivered, fighting to survive. I began to see an inner reserve in him that surpassed what I had believed he possessed.

While Dave was in the oxygen tent, the hospital sometimes bent their strict rules and let me stay the night, folded into a chair by his bed. I grew more and more haggard and worn out as time went on, never getting enough sleep.

Time seemed suspended as I waited for Dave to make progress, dreading to receive the report that he had not made it. Because of this, I always arrived at the hospital filled with anxiety, never knowing what I would encounter. I was stuck in a whirlpool, going round and round, powerless to get out.

The days dragged slowly by. It was now a week since Dave had caught pneumonia, and he still hung on to the edge of life, fighting each day to live another. Through it all, friends and family prayed for him, which was a source of comfort for me.

As I sat by Dave each day, I began to remember things he had done before the fire. He'd loved singing the old Canadian national anthem, "God Save the Queen." I thought about the time two years earlier when we'd gone to the school that Keir and Kimberly attended across the street from our house. There was a general assembly in the gym and we squeezed into the packed room along with all the students, teachers, and a few parents. At the end of the assembly, the national anthem was sung. The students sang softly, melodically, their voices rising and falling, blending together perfectly. As I remembered this, I could almost hear the voices of those children and adults joined together:

> *God save our gracious Queen*
> *Long live our noble Queen,*
> *God save the Queen:*
> *Send her victorious,*

Happy and glorious,
Long to reign over us:
God save the Queen.

That morning, I got caught up in the singing and it took me a while before I tuned into the atrocious sound hovering on the periphery of my hearing. Looking to my right, I saw Dave, mouth wide open, blaring at the top of his lungs, singing a song of his own. He was standing on a chair and we were near the front of the auditorium, so everyone was looking at him. I was so embarrassed.

Later that evening while I watched Dave brushing his teeth, he took up the refrain from the assembly earlier that day. He had a cup of water in his hand, rinsing his mouth, when suddenly he raised the cup up high in his right hand and declared, "God bless the Queen, stinky and glorious!"

He was only three at the time and it was too funny. Though I tried, I was unable to keep a straight face. I burst out laughing.

The memory brought a smile to my lips. I had so few smiles in those days. With the smile came tears, for after each brief shaft of sunshine in my heart I was jolted back to the gravity of Dave's present situation.

On the tenth day of Dave's pneumonia, the doctor permitted himself a slight smile as he told me things were looking hopeful.

CHAPTER 7

. . . .

KEIR GOES HOME

October–Mid-November

Roberta

D ave's condition continued to look hopeful, and I still remember the day the doctors proclaimed him out of danger! He was on his way to being well, a huge relief for me. Catastrophes, like the pneumonia, were almost too much for my heart to take. Dave's bout of pneumonia was particularly bad and came with a high fever, but the doctors were finally saying that the fever was down.

Things were looking up again. He began eating and drinking well and his skin grafts were all taking satisfactorily. His eyes, with grafted lids, were finally unwrapped. The bandages that had been on for weeks were removed and, although he may have needed one more graft to his eyelids, everything seemed to be going well.

In addition to Dave's good news, Keir was to be coming home soon. When I told Grandma, we danced around the kitchen with joy.

Once Dave became a little stronger, he began going for physical therapy and started daily trips to an immersion pool, where the thick, hardened skin of his upper body was scraped off. Originally this was done in the operating room because of the large amounts of dead skin that needed to be removed. Now that there wasn't much left, it was done in the pool. It was a very painful process. Watching all the difficult procedures Dave had to go through left a constant lump in my throat. It was hard for me to watch my baby boy enduring all this.

I wished I could go through the operations and pain for him. I felt like the physical pain would have been easier for me than the psychological pain of watching him go through it. Sadly, though, Dave had to go through this alone. But I was there by his side every time he cleared another tough hurdle. I was there to cuddle him, hold him, sing and talk to him, and let him know I was by his side.

Dave was bathed regularly in a pool. He was rolled into the pool room on a stretcher, then transferred to a pallet suspended by cables from a machine high above. The machine then swung him over the center of the pool and lowered him in until he was submerged up to his neck. His feet were pointed down towards the bottom of the pool, where he lay in a reclined position. At this point, a couple of nurses got into the water with him and started to scrape off the dead skin from his chest, back, head, face, hands, and arms. When he needed a break from this intense procedure, they would get him to move his limbs around to keep them limber. I only watched this procedure once. It was too hard for me to watch Dave go through this, alternately screaming and crying.

Dave didn't let the baths dampen his spirits, though. After each session, the machine lifted him out of the pool and the operator guided the pallet over to the stretcher, gently lowering him down. The nurses were there to fold him in warm blankets, and he promptly fell asleep.

Dave began talking more and more, remaining a wonderful kid through it all. The nurses were impressed and remarked on several occasions how refreshing they found it that Dave could remain a happy little boy through all the hardships. After several weeks of these sessions, he became more active and inquisitive.

One day, after he had been allowed to visit with Keir, he asked me about Kimberly. It cut to the core of my heart.

"Where's Kimberly, Mom? She hasn't visited me."

"Was she burned, too?"

"When is she coming to visit me? I miss her."

"I wanna see her."

"Everyone else has come to visit. How come she hasn't?"

I tried to choke back the tears. My daughter Kimberly was gone and the wound was still raw. I was in anguish! I rushed from the room with sobs coming from deep within me, deep heaving sobs that I could not stop.

As I rushed from the room, memories of Kimberly flooded my mind. I saw her as a young girl, getting up early while Daddy and I were still in bed and coming into our room with her teddy bear. She'd leave her bear with me to keep me company while she went off to play downstairs.

She was such a sweet girl and very protective of her family. A few years earlier, Ellis had been sick one day, leaving me to explain to Kimberly what was wrong with Daddy.

"He has the flu bug, Kimberly."

She came right back with, "Well, I'll stomp that bug with my shoe!"

The memory brought a smile to my face and a bit of pain seeped out of my heart. I realized then that I wasn't the only one hurting. Dave missed Kimberly, too, and his heart must have ached to see her again, just as mine did. It was time that I told him what had happened.

When I composed myself I went back into the room, I sat by Dave and told him how Kimberly had died in the fire. He looked so sad that I had to stay with him longer than usual that day. Even after he heard the news, Dave managed to remain his happy, fun-loving self. I hoped that throughout his life he would be able to maintain a young heart in order to regain some of the childhood he was losing during this time.

The doctors had been talking of sending Keir across the street to the children's ward of the Glenrose Rehabilitation Hospital to complete his recovery once he was released. But when his release date was extended, they kept him at the Royal Alex until no further work remained. He was then released to live at home.

Dave's condition was still serious, as the doctors still needed to do a lot of work on his body to make him well. Dave was in and out of the operating room, sometimes just to get a wound rebandaged. His chest, arms, back, and face were almost healed. His head and hands still needed plenty of work.

Dr. Strazinsky, a second plastic surgeon, was in the process of taking over from Dr. Timmons to complete the skin grafts. Dr. Strazinsky had just finished his training in plastic surgery and therefore was aware of the latest treatments for burns. The eyelids and ears that he had constructed for Dave, however, were not lasting. He had lost both in the fire and Dr. Strazinsky had tried several times to reconstruct them.

Nonetheless, Dave had become a good little fighter and remained in good spirits. Grandma and I got him a record with songs that he knew, including "The Little Drummer Boy." The day we brought it in, Dave sat in a chair most of the morning keeping time to the music with his little feet. I thoroughly enjoyed watching him tap his feet and wiggle his toes to the beat of the music. He was transfixed with the music, and I was mesmerized by his tapping feet.

Dave was put on a high-protein diet in the fall to make up for the weight he'd lost while fighting off pneumonia. A tube had been reinserted in his stomach for feeding purposes. The feedings were spaced every four hours, around the clock. It was a bold move to try and put some weight on him; his body was just skin and bones.

Because Dave was doing so much better, Keir was allowed to see him. They had wonderful visits together. Keir was still very much concerned about his little brother.

They had fun by thinking up riddles for each other, something that Keir had learned from all his time spent with Grandma.

I was so impressed with how well Dave was doing. He was becoming more active, moving his arms, wrists, and hands on a regular basis. He seemed to enjoy it and the nurses loved watching him happily doing what they normally had to coerce him to do.

After the feeding tube was removed again, we were back to feeding him by hand. The doctors were confident that something could be created to assist Dave in feeding himself. That was many months away, though. Following the intense feeding, Dave's weight was measured and he weighed in at a mere thirty-two pounds. He was still skin and bones and looked very thin. His sixth birthday was four months away.

Dave was scheduled for surgery again the following Monday for skin grafts on his head, back, and chest. It was slow going, because he had very few suitable places to take skin from now, since all unburned areas of his body had already been used many times. The skin could only be taken from places that hadn't been burned, and once taken from these spots the areas then had to heal and grow new skin before they could be used again.

Dave asked the doctors about his hands and they told him there was no infection in them. There was, however, infection in other parts of his body and the doctors were working on those areas at present. His hands, for the time being, were wrapped in pig skin; this was to keep them moist and keep the air off to avoid infection. Human skin would normally have been used for this, but when that ran out pig skin was a viable alternative. The doctors planned to keep his hands wrapped until they could do some work on them.

One day that fall, Grandma came to me. I could tell from her face that there was something she wanted to talk about, but she did not know how to bring it up. She finally spoke, telling me that she was considering leaving when Keir was allowed to return home. I felt sick to my stomach as the words hit home. I tried to put on a brave face, even though I couldn't even think straight.

We discussed it at length and I told her that if she had to leave, I would be okay. She seemed to sense how I was really feeling, though, and decided that she'd stay as long as needed. I had no more recollection of what else was said. She later told me that I'd turned green when she brought up the subject. That would explain the sick feeling I got.

The weather started getting cooler, so we gathered together some winter clothes for Grandma. I lent her a coat and she went shopping, buying a winter hat, gloves, lined boots, and winter slacks. The spring and summer clothes she had brought with her back in May were okay for fall, but she needed hardier clothing for our harsh Edmonton winters.

A short while later, an idea began forming in my mind. *What if we can have Dave home for Christmas?* Then we could have both boys home. It would depend on whether Dave was healthy enough. I discussed it with Grandma, who agreed that we would have to see.

The more the thought germinated, though, the more I realized that Christmas would be quite somber if Dave wasn't home with us. Surely the doctors would at least let him come home for the day.

I knew Dave's health was still a big concern, and I didn't want to jeopardize it for the sake of the rest of the family. I brought up the subject with the doctors, with the understanding that they would consider it and we would wait and see how Dave's health progressed. We were still more than two months away from Christmas.

Keir didn't get to go home in mid-September as the doctors had originally planned, but ended up home at the end of October. The day he was to go home, he was so excited that he bounced around non-stop. Nothing could dampen his spirits. It was a cool day, so we dressed him warmly and packed him in the car to go home.

Within days of Keir going home, the nurses began talking about getting Dave up and walking. His legs were so weak from lying in bed all those months that the muscles would have to be strengthened.

"We'll do it a little at a time," one of the nurses said. "A few seconds at first, then we'll work at it over time until we are up to a minute. We'll stand him up, and when we do this the blood will rush to his legs where it hasn't been circulating for well over five months now. He won't be accustomed to having so much blood rushing through the veins in his legs. It will be very painful, so don't be surprised when he screams. It will be unbearable at first."

Unbearable? Wasn't everything Dave was going through unbearable? But I knew he would handle it just as he had handled everything else. I was so proud of my young son.

The day finally came when the nurses told me they would start standing Dave up. I wanted to make sure I was there. It was to be right after breakfast the next day, which was served at the crack of seven. I hoped to be at the hospital by eight o'clock, just after he finished eating. The nurses assured me that they would not start until I arrived.

On the bus ride to the hospital the next day, I remembered what the nurses had told me the day before—they would hold Dave up for just a few seconds and then gradually get him used to having the blood flow through his legs again.

When I arrived at the hospital, I hurried to Dave's room.

CHAPTER 8

LEARNING TO WALK AGAIN

Mid-November–December 31

Roberta

Dave was sitting up in bed; his breakfast was finished, and as always he was happy to see me. I had a twinge in my heart as I saw his face. How I wished the hospital would allow me to stay until he was asleep each night to make life a little less tough on him.

Two nurses entered the room, joining the one already there. They told Dave that they were just going to lift him for just a few seconds and that it would hurt a lot.

"Are you ready, Dave?" one of them asked. "Do you need more time?"

Dave shook his head, and in his high, thin voice managed to say, "I don't think so."

The nurses moved quickly and purposefully. They slid Dave to the end of the bed and let him dangle his feet over the edge. Then, quick as a flash, with one nurse on either side of him, they lifted him to an upright position, his feet barely resting on the floor.

No sooner was he in the air than he started screaming. I was transfixed by the scene before me: Dave held upright by two nurses, his mouth wide open, blaring out a scream that went right to the core of my being.

Then, as quickly as it started, it was over and Dave was being tucked back in bed where he promptly fell asleep.

The nurses continued to stand him up once a day from that point on. The pain was at first unbearable, the blood rushing into his legs every time he stood up. So the nurses only held him up until the pain became too much, and then they would quickly put him back in bed.

Dave had not been walking for about five months and it seemed he had forgotten how. This was not surprising since he was only five and had spent so many months now lying in bed, immobile, unconscious, and drugged. He would not have forgotten had he been older. Not only did he now need to strengthen his legs, he had to learn how to walk all over again.

It took over a couple of weeks before Dave could bear to stand up without screaming in pain. Then, when he could handle it, he practiced walking with the help of the nurses. One day he tried walking by himself: steadying himself with his hands, he walked along the side and then around the edge of the bed. From there he could reach the chair at the foot of his bed, then crawl into it. It was about seven steps in total. This chair was so large that, with his legs straight in front of him, his little feet hung over the edge.

Dave practiced walking day after day until he finally took some steps without the support of the bed. He tottered, regained his balance, and made it to the chair.

The day came when the nurses told him he was going to walk to the door of his room. Nurses from all over the hospital came to witness him take this awesome step forward. What a fighter he was turning out to be! What a moment it was when Dave reached the door and the nurses clapped in excitement for him!

It was now only weeks until Christmas and I conferred with the doctors to see if Dave could come home for the holidays. They were less skeptical than they'd been the last time we talked on this subject.

"Well, Mrs. Hammer," Dr. Strazinsky said, "if Dave keeps progressing the way he is now, we should be able to see our way clear to let him go home for the holidays."

I could not wait to have Dave home and away from the hospital for a spell. I was so sick of the drab walls, the hospital sounds and smells, and the dreary feeling of sickness all about. Even having Dave home for Christmas Day would have been a boost, but as Keir reminded me, "If he can't come home, we'll bring Christmas to him!"

Dave was still learning how to walk again and I saw intense concentration on his face as he tried to recall: *How did I used to walk? Why is it so tough now?* The one thing I noticed was that he didn't seem to remember or realize he needed to bend his knees when he walked. He was walking stiff-legged, which wasn't quite natural.

Dave was still very weak and got tired quickly, so relearning to walk was a very slow process. He slept a lot of the day but would be awake for meals, take small walks in the morning, stay awake until after lunch, then sleep the afternoon through. Grandma and I would come in the morning and stay until the noon meal, then would leave and return again in the early evening for supper. After supper, Dave usually stayed awake for a few hours and then fell asleep for the night. We would have to leave in the evening before he fell asleep, but I didn't like leaving him like that.

Before long, Christmas was only two weeks away. The doctors decided that Dave could go home for the holidays! This would be the ultimate test. If Dave came back healthy, it would be a sign that he would make it, that he would survive this horrible tragedy and push on to see what he could make of himself.

With the knowledge that Dave would likely be home for Christmas, we started preparing the house for his arrival. We had to make sure the whole place was clean as a whistle so Dave would not catch anything. Grandma, Keir (who had been home now for some weeks), and I scrubbed walls, floors, carpets, and made sure all Dave's linens were washed and his room sanitized. It was a lot of work and we were all tired by the time it was complete.

Ellis surprised us by dropping in on a Saturday and helping us with the cleaning. He brought joy to the house by clowning around the whole time. I hadn't laughed for quite some time and my stomach muscles didn't know how to respond. They sure were sore the next day. It was great for Keir, too, who enjoyed having his dad around for the whole day.

Grandma and I went Christmas shopping one cold winter day, the snow thick upon the ground. We came away with some fun presents for the boys and a new scarf for Ellis. We split up at one point to get something for each other so that it would be a surprise on Christmas Day.

Finally, the day came. On a chilly December 24, we wheeled Dave out in a wheelchair to our running car. Ellis was waiting behind the wheel. We took Dave out of the wheelchair all bundled up in winter garb and sat him gently in the backseat. Once we had carefully buckled him in so as not to hurt him, we were ready to roll. We headed for home.

When Keir had come home, he'd changed the whole dynamic of the household. It was the same having Dave home again. He wasn't awake much of the day, but when he was his peals of laughter could be heard through the entire house. It had been seven months since the fire, but during that time Dave had not lost his sense of humor.

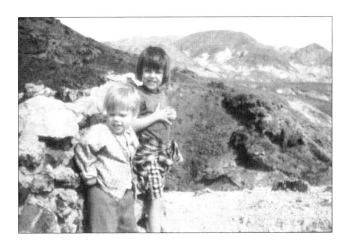

Keir and Kimberly

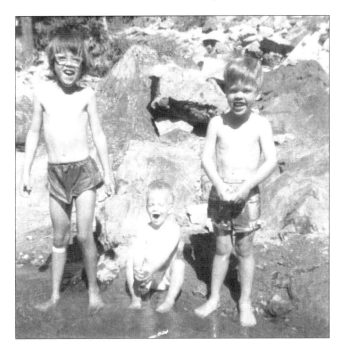

Kimberly, Dave and Keir

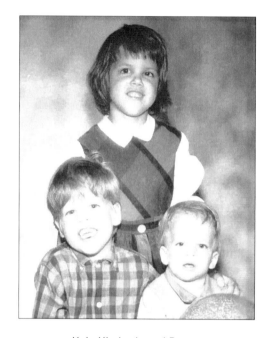

Keir, Kimberly and Dave

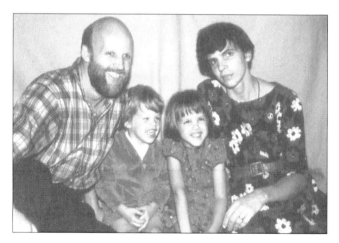

(Left to right) Dad, Keir, Kimberly and Mom

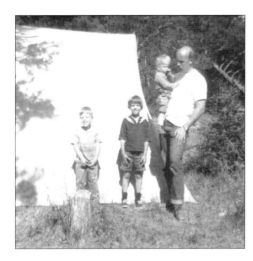

(Left to right)
Keir, Kimberly,
Dave and Dad

(Left to right) Keir,
Kimberly and Dave

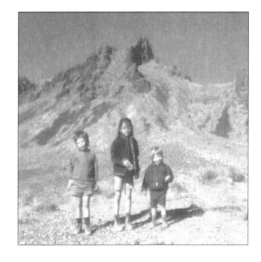

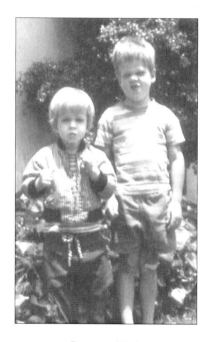

Dave and Keir

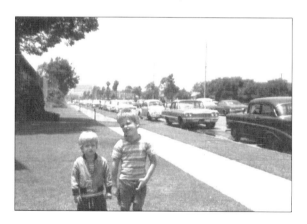

Dave and Keir

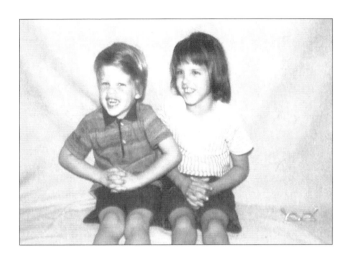

Keir and Kimberly

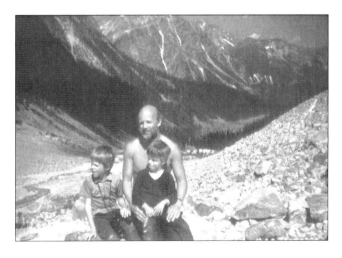

Keir, Dad and Dave

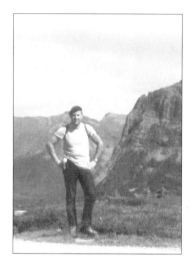

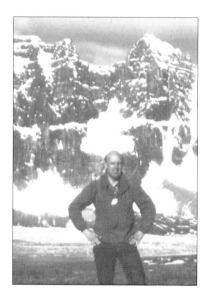

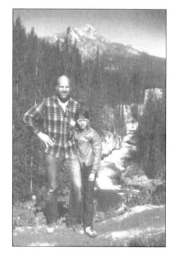

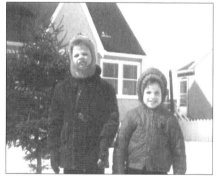

(Top left and right) Dad
(Left) Dad and Kimberly
(Right) Keir and Dave

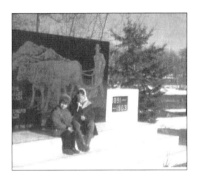

Dave and Kimberly

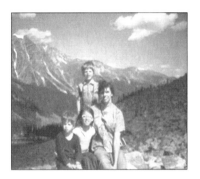

Dave, Kimberly, Keir and Mom

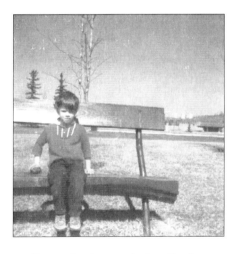

Dave, about a year before the fire

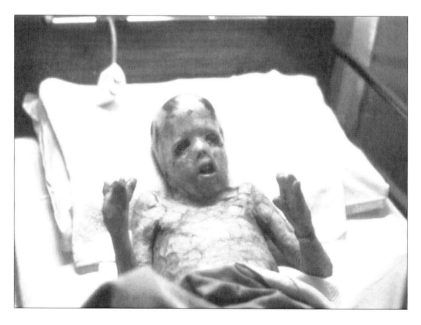

Dave, 14 months after the fire, and
after 3 consecutive operations

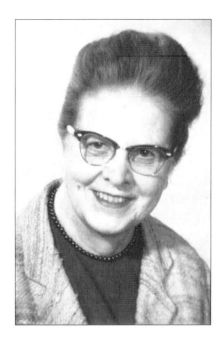

(Above) Grandma
(Right) Mom

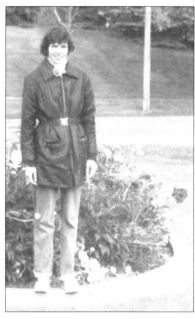

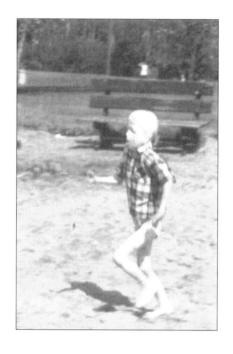

(Above & right) Dave

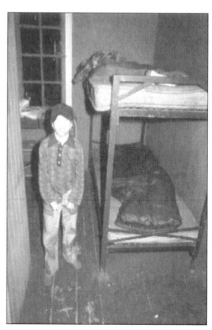

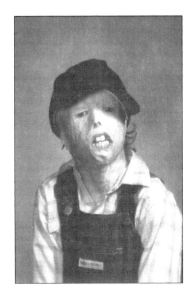

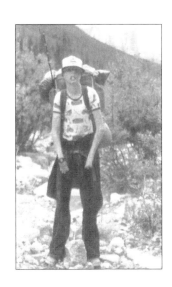

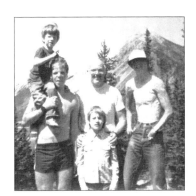

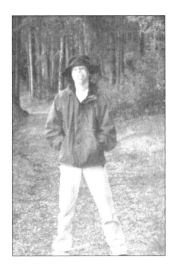

(Top Right) Dave on a backbacking trip
(Bottom Left) Evan, Keir, Shauna, Dad and Dave

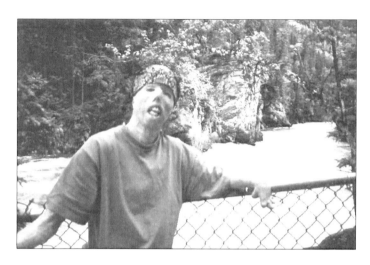

Dave in the mountains

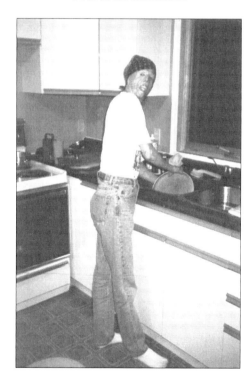

Dave doing dishes

CHAPTER 9

THE TURNING POINT

Dave

You may be wondering why I haven't yet explained the cause of the fire. The whos, whats, wheres, whens, hows, and whys seemed to come in segments after the night of the accident. Our first priority in this tragedy was healing. Understanding followed later.

In trying to understand and piece together the events of the fateful night of the fire, I spoke to neighbors and any witnesses I could find. I also tried to track down police reports, coroner's reports, and legal documents. Unfortunately, some documents had been destroyed since the fire many years ago and I was not able to locate some of the witnesses, but from everyone I spoke to, and what I was able to read, I have pieced together how that night must have unfolded.

What follows is a third-person narrative of the events of that night.

*   *   *

George had a bad feeling. He and two friends—Carl and Tom—had dozens of firecrackers, setting them off as they wandered the streets. The hour was late when they arrived in the vicinity of their homes. George lived just a block away and Tom only two blocks away. They were close to Carl's home when they spotted a tent in the backyard two doors down.

"This is Garry's house," Tom whispered.

They crept up quietly, able to hear the slow breathing of people asleep inside the tent.

Tom smiled. "Let's give him a scare!"

George looked at Tom, trying to see if he were serious, but couldn't make his face out in the darkness.

"Are you serious? We don't even know if he's in here! Maybe it's his younger sister," George hissed.

"Quit being a crybaby, George!" Tom's face was hard. He began crawling around to the far side of the tent, Carl following right behind him.

George watched them go, and a moment later followed. When he was around the tent, he saw Tom by the door.

"Pull the tent pegs," Tom said. Carl and George crawled around the tent, pulling out the pegs as quickly as they could. The top of the tent started to sag and sway when they finished.

When they returned to the area where Tom was, he was holding a number of firecrackers in one hand and a pack of matches in the other. When he saw that Carl and George were back from their job, he extended his hand with the firecrackers toward them.

"Hold these," Tom whispered.

Carl obediently reached out to take them, but George stubbornly kept his hands by his sides. Tom opened the pack of matches, tore one from the group, and lit it. Then, taking the firecrackers from Carl, he lit a couple and threw them into the area of the tent entrance.[1] That's when George started getting a bad feeling. The tent had been breached. They all bolted to the nearby alley.

They waited and a few seconds later the firecrackers went off. They didn't hear anyone stirring in the tent and no one stuck their head out the door to see what was going on. The boys left, chalking it up to a failed practical joke.

As they neared the corner, a police car cruised by, braked, and stopped. Two policemen got out. The boys scattered, running back down the alley in the direction from which they had come. Tom ran towards a school bus that was parked nearby. He rolled under it, and as George ran after him he saw Tom place a string of a dozen firecrackers behind the rear wheel. Then Tom threw another string of firecrackers further under the bus.

That's all George saw before a policeman caught him. Tom peeked out from under the bus to see what was happening, but the two policemen had George and Carl by then.

"You can come out from under the bus, son," one of the officers told Tom. Once the boys were all standing side by

---

1   Based on a report by the coroner's office, written a month after the fire regarding the ban of firecracker sales.

side, the police had them empty out their pockets. When they had finished, there was a pile of firecrackers on the pavement, two dozen in all.

*   *   *

A short time later…

Scott jumped out of bed, then ran downstairs and out the back door, right behind his wife. He could see the west side of the tent engulfed in flames: fingers of fire running up to the roof.

His wife Bernice ran after Kat, who had just gotten out of the tent with her pajamas on fire. As Bernice ran past the tent, trying to catch Kat, the roof collapsed. Scott couldn't bear the thought of the children inside suffering, so he ran towards the tent.

He leaped into the fire, most of the roof having already burned by the time he got there, and grabbed Keir. He picked him up and threw him out onto the grass. Looking back in the tent he saw Dave, the youngest neighbor boy, only five years old. Bending over, he scooped him into his arms and carried him gingerly out of the tent. The entire time, Scott's feet were being licked and burned by the fire he bravely stood in. He looked back in the fire to see if there were any others he could spot, but he could see nothing but flames.

Scott turned his attention towards his wife and daughter just as Keir ran past him, his pajamas burning brightly. He was about to chase Keir when his wife beat him to it. Having just finished extinguishing the flames on her daughter, Bernice took off after Keir.[2]

* * *

In the wee hours of the night, Roberta was jarred awake. There was an incessant pounding on the back door downstairs and the doorbell kept ringing. Her heart leapt into her throat.

What's going on here?

She knew something was wrong. Flinging on her bathrobe, she hurried down the stairs and flung open the door. The scene that met her eyes was more than her mind could comprehend.

She saw the tent next door engulfed in fire. In truth, all she could see were flames, but she just knew it was the tent burning.

Keir was standing in front of her. Something was wrong with his hands; they looked like they were melting. The skin was dripping off them and he was trying to catch it, sort of like a juggling act. His pajamas were rags with burn holes all over and his hair was gone.

She looked next door again and saw a little boy, his upper body—stomach, chest, arms, neck, head, and face—completely black from the fire. His pajama shirt was in tatters. By his size, she knew it was Dave.

My God, what have I done?

In a panic, she ran towards the three-foot high wooden

---

2 Bernice has no recollection of catching up to Keir until he reached his house, but on the other hand Keir recalls being knocked to the ground three times. The first may have been when he was thrown out of the tent onto the grass, and he may have fallen while he ran.

fence separating her from the yard next door. Her adrenaline kicking in, she vaulted over the fence in a single leap. When she landed on the grass on the other side, she looked around to find her daughter Kimberly.

She saw Scott's daughter, Kat, thankfully alive. But she couldn't find her daughter. Seeing Bernice, she asked where Kimberly was but received no response.

Roberta walked toward the tent, but there was nothing left of it anymore; it had all burned up. Instead she saw two bodies, lying motionless where the tent had been, black and lifeless. Her heart leapt into her throat as she realized it was Kimberly and Beth, the girl from two doors down.

This can't be happening!

She thought she was dreaming. Her only daughter, Kimberly, couldn't be dead. She just couldn't! She felt tears streaming down her face and knew it was no dream she could wake up from. There was no going back to what *had* been, either. She knelt there, beside Kimberly's lifeless body, and let out gut-wrenching cries.

*   *   *

Across the parking lot were a string of duplexes where a young boy and his parents lived. The boy woke in the middle of the night to use the bathroom. He woke his mom, Jean, when he crept upstairs. Jean saw the reflection of flickering light on her bedroom wall.

"Something is happening out there," she said, shaking Roy, her husband, awake.

"It's just kids playing with fire," he replied.

"No," she said. "I think people are on fire!"

They quickly got up, dressed, and ran over to help. At that point, Bernice was trying to lead Roberta away from the fire. Keir and Dave were lying on the grass, screaming. Roy acted quickly and drove everyone to the hospital, since it would have taken too long for an ambulance to arrive. None of the passengers recalled who travelled in the car that night. All their bodies had gone into shock to deal with the horror.

DAVE

CHAPTER 10

AWAKE!

Dave, Age 5

When I first recall waking up in the hospital, I was flat on my back. I think it was sometime in September, over three months after the fire, but I have no way to confirm this. When I opened my eyes, the first thing I saw was the ceiling. Sunbeams played across its surface and my gaze followed the dancing beams down the walls. This world of sunshine was so bright and refreshing after my world of darkness.

My nose itched and I wanted to scratch it. In fact, I tried to scratch it. I lifted my hand and saw that it was all wrapped up in bandages. Then my brain registered more than the itch on my nose and I realized that my whole body itched. I searched the room with my eyes to see if there was anyone to help. I saw no one, so I promptly went to sleep and the itching faded away.

When I awoke again, I was at peace. It felt as if I had awakened from a very long sleep and was incredibly refreshed. Everything looked bright and cheery in my room that morning. Colors looked brighter and more fantastic than I remembered.

My mom and dad walked into the room a little later. When they saw that I was awake, they both smiled.

"Hi Mommy and Daddy," I said, looking from one to the other. Then my eyes settled on my dad. "Will you read me another story, Daddy?" I asked, my voice filled with longing.

"Of course, son." His face beamed with pleasure and I closed my eyes with a sigh of happiness.

He told me about Mom moving Keir, Kimberly, and me a couple weeks before the fire and he drew me a picture of our home there.

As he talked, I remembered that Dad and Mom had split up and that was why we moved. Dad stayed in Edmonton. Eventually I drifted off to sleep, content with the sound of my dad's voice close by.

When I awoke next, it was dark in the room and I could hear nurses walking up and down the hall.

"Anything you need, Dave?"

I jumped, not realizing anyone was near. "Yes, please," I rasped, my throat dry from my sleep. "Could I have some apple juice and something to eat?"

"Sure thing, honey. I'll see what the cook has. Be back in a minute." Then the nurse was gone, off in search of a snack.

A short while later, she reappeared with a silver tray with two glasses on it—one glass of apple juice and one of milk. Beside them sat a plate with a big slice of chocolate cake. The nurses were always eager to run down to the kitchen to see what the cook had for me. Even down in the kitchen they knew who I was and did their best to find me goodies to eat. They even made cakes especially with me in mind, knowing I loved them so much.

The nurse grinned happily as she set the tray on my bedside table. "Here you are, Dave. The cook made this cake a little earlier today, just for you." She took a few steps toward the door then turned, paused, and looked at me a moment. "Do you want some help eating, Dave?"

I nodded and she quickly pulled a chair up to my bed and started feeding me the cake while I happily slurped the milk in between bites. The apple juice I saved for later.

She told me stories of her boyfriend and her plans for the future while she fed me. I didn't catch all she said because I was concentrating on the delicious chocolate cake. It was enough that she was sharing from her heart and taking me into her confidence. It filled me with a warmth I had not experienced before. I was very content.

After I had been awake for a couple of months, the doctors told the kitchen staff that I needed a lot of calories. They tracked down my mom to find out what I liked.

"Milkshakes and cake!" she told them. Those were my favorites! From then on, the cook made those things special for me. When I asked for something to eat after all the meals had been served for the day, the nurses would run off to the kitchen to see what the cook had.

My mom, dad, and grandma told me numerous times how happy they were that I was awake more. I knew they loved having me awake when they came to visit, but I would find out soon enough that I was not so happy to be awake! The many operations in the months that followed became a terror to me.

Needles were painful things for me. The doctors would always say, "This will prick just a bit," or, "This will feel like a mosquito bite." But it never felt like a little prick; it felt as if someone was pinching me as hard as they could. I came to dread needles. I needed time to ready myself for them but was rarely given that time. I would have to beg and plead to prepare myself. I'm sure the funniest picture of me, if it had been caught on film, would have been when I crawled around my bed at top speed with my pajama bottoms down, crying, "Just a sec! Just a sec!"

As a child, it took me a lot longer to brace myself for the pain than it did when I became an adult. At least one needle preceded every operation, so I dreaded operations. A needle would usually be administered before I left my room, in order to calm me down, and another in the operating room to put me under before the operation. I was so terrified of needles that in the operating room I would beg for them to use the gas mask to put me under, which they did many times, but only if I asked. Sometimes the doctors already had the needle prepared, so it was too late.

After the operation, I felt a different kind of pain. It was the pain of a wound healing. The area would be tender and sore to the touch, and as it healed it itched. When the time came for the dressing to be removed, it was very painful.

This pain, though, was nothing compared to the emotional pain I underwent prior to each operation. The waiting was excruciating.

I expected needles every second of every minute from the time I woke up until the day was over. A nurse would push a cart down the hall to administer medicine or take blood. In the cart were glass vials, and they all rattled together as the cart rolled down the hall, stopping at each room on that day's list. That sound was a terror to me and I was happiest when it was far out of earshot.

Sometimes I would lie in terror for hours, waiting to hear the nurse coming to give me my needle. On the days that the cart passed by my room, I knew from experience that it would not be back anytime soon. The easiest part was after I had received a needle. Then I could relax and breathe easy for the rest of the day, knowing the needle cart would not stop at my room again until the next day.

It's a terrible thing to go through the most painful and horrible ordeal of your life as a five-year-old. My family wasn't always able to be there when I needed them. It just wasn't possible for them to be with me around the clock for such a long period of time.

Now, as an adult, the smells I encounter walking through a hospital bring back such vivid memories that my heart will start to pound rapidly, my stomach will flip, making me nauseous, and I'll have difficulty breathing. It's as if I were swept back into the horrors of the hospital, as a five-year-old. It has only been in the past five years that those reactions have subsided. I still prefer to avoid hospitals, though.

The orderlies and nurses, as a general rule, tried to lessen my suffering as much as they were able. One orderly, knowing how terrified I was of getting a needle in the operating room, wanted to take me right in there himself so he could be there with me. When it was time for my operation, he wheeled me down in a wheelchair, but when we got to the door of the O.R. they would not let him in, because his clothes were not sterile and it would compromise the sterile environment inside.

I really appreciated his attempt to come in with me, but I knew that no one was allowed inside, not even my mom. This was one area that I always went into by myself, having to face the terror completely and utterly alone. Sure, the doctors and nurses were there, but no one who could face these fears with me.

One day after an operation, I woke up and felt something attached to my toe. I looked up at the wall and saw a half-filled bag of red liquid hanging from a metal pole. I could see a tube running to a needle in my big toe. I lay there for a long time, just watching the contents of the bag drip down to my foot.

When my mom came into the room a little while later, the curiosity bubbled up in me.

"What's in that bag?" I asked.

She turned to look. "Oh! That? Well, that's blood. The doctors took so many blood tests, Dave, and with so much blood out of your body, they need to put some back into you."

I tried to remember getting enough blood tests to fill a quart-sized bag. I couldn't remember that many.

*   *   *

I had to learn to walk again after my months and months of lying inactive in bed. My leg muscles were wasting away because of lack of use. In addition to weak legs, my young age and months spent in bed meant that I'd forgotten how to walk.

To get me back up and around, the nurses came in and got me up on my feet. I didn't stand on the floor but was held up as my feet dangled free. As the blood rushed into my legs at full force, the pain was so intense that I screamed. As time went on, the feeling lessened from intense pain to a tingling sensation.

Once I reached this stage, I was held up and supported by two nurses with my feet barely on the floor until, in time, I could hold my full weight on my legs. Then I would take a few steps with a nurse on either side to hold me up.

Eventually, I was able to balance with the help of the nurses. I tried walking by holding on to something for support. I began to set small goals for myself to try to walk to. The first one I chose was a chair at the foot of my bed. It was a chore to cover even that short of distance. I did it using the bed for balance, walking along with one hand resting on it.

Once I had mastered that, I tried walking to the chair without holding anything for support. I wobbled a little, then gritted my teeth and concentrated hard. I made it! I felt secure knowing I could always grab onto the bed if I lost my balance.

The day came when the nurses told me it was time to try walking to the door of my hospital room. It was a very long way for me. Getting to the chair had been a struggle in itself, but now that I had mastered that distance, I felt I was ready to try a longer distance.

The day of my walk arrived and nurses started to gather from far and wide; word of my walk had spread. I crawled out of bed all swathed in bandages, wearing white socks, a white hospital gown, and white bandages on my arms—I was covered in white as I took my first step. I started into the open with nothing to hold onto. The door looked so far away.

A bunch of nurses were already watching me and one of them yelled, "Here he comes!" More nurses came running down the hall from every corner of the ward.

They filled the room, leaving me a path to the door, a path wide enough that I could not grab onto them for support. I could hear more nurses rushing down the hallway to see me walk as I took step after step.

The door looked so far away and my steps didn't seem to bring me much closer. Halfway there, my strength was starting to fail. I thought I'd collapse from fatigue before I got there. Then, from somewhere deep inside me, determination rose up, pressing me on, unwilling to fail.

Suddenly the door seemed much closer and I felt eager to reach my goal. Shuffling on, step by step, I could almost reach the door frame. That was my goal…I'd stop there. With one step to go, I reached out and rested my bandaged hand against the door frame. The nurses' cheering drowned out the sound of the blood pounding in my ears from my exertion.

I was suddenly enveloped in the warm embraces of the nurses and they carried me back to my bed where I fell asleep, contented with my achievement. It was only about fifteen to twenty feet, but to me it was like walking a mile.

I took a longer walk next time. The nurses urged me to walk to the door again, but I looked them defiantly in the face and declared, "No! I want to walk to the playroom!" And I did! The playroom was out my door and quite a ways down the hall…certainly a much longer walk for me.

The more I walked, the stronger my legs became, and soon I was running up and down the halls, much to the delight of the nurses. That's when they told me that I wasn't bending my knees when I walked. Yet I was going up and down the stairs with no problem. They showed me how their knees bent when they walked. I would try to imitate them, but I always bent my knee after I had taken the step, not while I was taking it.

I practiced and practiced. Then one day when I wasn't trying so hard to figure things out, I did it. I took the perfect step and I never looked back.

As winter approached, I wrote a letter to Santa and gave it to one of the nurses to mail to the North Pole. Little did I know that she passed it on all right—to my parents. There was only one request in the letter: I wanted an SSP Racer, a popular toy car at the time.

An SSP had only two wheels, one in the front of the car and one in the back, both balanced like on a bicycle. A plastic cord with teeth on it was inserted into a hole in the middle of the toy car and quickly pulled, which caused the wheels to spin fast. Then, with the wheels spinning, the car would race away once placed on the floor. The speed at which it traveled kept the car balanced on its two wheels.

Christmas drew near and I was scheduled to go home, but a few days before I was to be taken home, Mom and Dad surprised me with an early present.

They made me close my eyes. When I opened my eyes, they got as big as saucers. It was an SSP! How had they known? I had sent my letter requesting it from Santa and hadn't told anyone else. I was so excited to have one!

The hospital halls were perfect for the SSP, because they were long and wide. My little car simply flew down them at incredible speeds. I liked to run down the hall after my SSP, my body bandaged, my head bandaged, my legs bandaged, my right arm sometimes in a sling after an operation, white socks on my feet, white undergarments, and my white hospital gown billowing out behind me.

CHAPTER 11

....

GLADYS

Dave, Age 5¾

The nurses had never seen me as happy as I was with my new toy and they never scolded me for playing with it. They even smiled occasionally when they found it underfoot at inappropriate times.

When Christmas arrived, I was whisked home by my mom, dad, and grandma. It was so much fun being at home that I ran all over the house hollering in delight at everything I saw.

I ran out of energy quickly and was tucked into bed in my own room where I slept soundly for hours. I felt like I slept away many days over Christmas.

My mom and dad were very concerned with my health. Both of them were quick to see if I needed anything; they never seemed to mind jumping up and getting me something. In fact, they seemed glad to do it. My dad, although still not living with us, came over every day during the holidays.

Before I knew it, my time at home was at an end and back to the hospital I went. I missed being at home where I knew I was safe and no one could come and hurt me. The hospital seemed a depressing place, especially compared to the warmth of being with my family.

My return to the hospital began a new series of sessions in some sort of pool which were, to put it quite simply, horrible but necessary. For each session, I was lowered into the pool on a sort of portable stretcher suspended from lines above. As soon as I was lowered into the water the top of the stretcher got hooked onto the wall of the pool. I would still be lying on the stretcher but my feet would be submerged in the water with my body suspended at a forty-five degree angle.

When I was in position, the nurses would go to work on me, scrubbing off the hard, damaged and dead skin with the tools of their trade. These would need to be abrasive enough to get the hard encrusted skin off. Underneath was new pink skin, which, once exposed, could breathe and flourish as it should.

These baths were horrible times for me. The pain was so intense that I screamed in agony during the whole process and then, once I was out, fell immediately asleep, exhausted from the ordeal. I would later wake up in my room. There was relief in being unconscious; I would learn that lesson over the next few years, and I would learn it well.

The nurses would always try to encourage me while I was in the pool by saying things like "We're almost finished, Dave" and "Hang in there, we're just about complete."

Thankfully they didn't say this all the way through the process or I would never have believed them. Instead they told me we were almost finished when it was true and I knew I only had to bear the pain for a few more moments. The nurses gave me a needle for the pain before these procedures, so at least the pain was lessened somewhat. Without the injection, I can't imagine what it would have been like.

I enjoyed most of the health care workers, from the nurses to the different therapists. Most of them treated me the same as they would anyone else. I imagine they treated me the same way they would have liked to be treated if they were in my shoes.

During this time, I underwent a lot of physical therapy (also known as physio) and occupational therapy (OT). The workers in these areas always passed on something useful to me, even if it was just advice here and there.

My hands were in bad shape. My thumbs were amputated to the first knuckle and my fingers to the second knuckle or lower, because dry gangrene had set in. It was certainly a struggle for me to learn to use my hands again after that. But I fought hard to try.

After my fingers were amputated, my hands were wrapped in pig skin to keep the stubs of my fingers moist. They were then left alone for months. The doctors unwrapped them later to see what they could do with what was left of my fingers.

The doctors preferred to wrap my hands in human skin, but this wasn't always available, so pig skin, the preferred substitute, was used. It would stay on seven to ten days before fresh skin was wrapped around my hands. In later years, the doctors had more options, but not at the beginning.

I needed to keep my legs, arms, shoulders, back, and neck mobile to slow the rate at which the skin grafts shrunk, otherwise the skin would tighten up so much that I would be very limited in my movements. To prevent this tightening, I did a lot of exercises, some of which I did in a swimming pool. I would wear a life jacket and be put in a heated swimming pool where I'd be instructed to move my arms around to get a full range of motion.

I didn't want to do this, because it hurt. I had to move my legs in these pool exercises because they were the main area where skin had been taken to transplant to my upper body. The physical therapist had to coax me to do my exercises. One such physical therapist, Mark, had to keep urging me, "Come on, Dave. Just try moving your arms a little bit."

"I can't!"

"Sure you can. Come on, just try to move a little tiny bit." I would move a bit and he would immediately say, "There you are! Now try a little more."

"No! I can't! It hurts!"

"I know it hurts, Dave, but just a little more. You're almost there."

I would do a bit more, and after I had done my movements long enough Mark would take me out of the pool and wrap me in a warm towel. He'd look me in the eye and say, "I told you, you could do it, Dave!"

I only stayed in the hospital about two months after Christmas. The doctors were so impressed that I had survived the holidays at home that they decided maybe I was further ahead than they thought. So they sent me across the street to the Glenrose Rehabilitation Hospital. The locals called it simply the "Glenrose." I was to be in the children's section of the hospital. This children's wing was adjoined to a school for students who were physically or mentally handicapped or challenged.

I was to live in the hospital ward and attend school. I was just across the street from the Royal Alex Hospital, where I had spent the last nine months. The two hospitals were joined by an underground tunnel, which I would be ferried back and forth through many times for operations. Then I'd be sent back across the street to the Glenrose.

Finally the day came for my hands to be taken out of the pig skin. I was taken over to the Royal Alex through the tunnel for surgery. Lying on a stretcher, I was wheeled through the grey, dimly lit tunnel with periodic lights in the ceiling. I didn't have much of a view lying flat on my back except those slivers of light.

When I woke up from the operation, Dr. Strazinsky, my plastic surgeon, was sitting beside my bed. I could tell he had been waiting to talk to me. As soon as I was alert enough, that's exactly what he did.

"Dave, your hands are all bandaged up right now because your fingers were stuck together and we had to cut them apart. Now, I placed a pin in each finger in order to keep your fingers straight so they don't curl up like they did in the pigskin. When it's time, I'll take them out."

I nodded, thinking he meant this would take place in another operation.

As if sensing this, he looked me in the eyes, and I saw a compassion there that I didn't always see in other hospital staff.

"Now, I want you to understand, Dave, that I'll take those pins out one at a time with a pair of pliers while you're awake. The pins won't hurt much coming out and it'll be over quickly, but they won't come out all the same day. Some days I'll take out one, or sometimes two."

I felt comforted by the fact that he told me they would come out quickly and wouldn't hurt much, and because of this I did not dread the days when it would happen.

When it was time for the first pin to come out, Dr. Strazinsky came in with a small pair of something that looked like needle-nose pliers. He pulled up a chair to my bed, took hold of the pin that extended out of my finger, about a quarter of an inch long, and with a quick yank it was out! I looked down at my little stub of a finger and watched a small drop of blood trickle out the end, but just as he promised, it didn't really hurt at all.

I stayed at the Royal Alex two months until all the pins were removed. Then I was sent back to the Glenrose.

At the Glenrose, straps were adapted for my hands to help me feed myself. Once the strap was attached to my hand by Velcro, I could insert a fork or spoon in it and feed myself. It was exciting for me to finally be able to do this and not have to rely on someone to help. I was happy to use the straps, but within a short time I became determined to figure out a way to feed myself without the use of them.

Learning to use my hands again was the most difficult of all the things I had to relearn. My fingers were now all one inch to one-and-half-inches long, except for my smallest baby finger, which was only half an inch long. My thumbs were one-and-a-half to two inches long. I had to work on them in physio, but even during my free time I was still learning to use them.

I struggled to be able to do everything I wanted to do. It was hard work and I had to learn to think outside the box. I couldn't just watch how someone else did it and then copy them; I had to learn my own way of doing things. Once I learned to use my hands, there was no going back.

In those early years after the fire, my hands were quite tender and handling things would hurt. I often thought through how to do something before I actually attempted it. It was less painful that way. Even at my young age of five, I was inclined to rely on my brain to figure things out rather than by trying. As my hands became less tender, I could try things over and over until I mastered them, but it was a highly frustrating road for me.

Shortly after Christmas, my grandma went back to her home and I missed her visits. But little did I know that soon I would have a new visitor.

As I lay recuperating in my room after one operation at the Royal Alex, a boy with a severe case of asthma was placed in the room next to mine. His mother, Gladys, saw me on one of her trips to visit her son and talked to my dad. Later she met my mom and asked what had happened to me.

Soon Gladys began visiting me when she came to see her son and we hit it off. I don't recall the first time I met her, but I'm sure we sparked to each other's sense of humor and wit.

Since Gladys was visiting me regularly, Mom would come in the morning and leave in the late afternoon so she could be home before Keir returned from school. Gladys would come right after she got off work and arrive around my suppertime.

A typical day in the hospital looked something like this:

7:00 AM: Rise and shine and have a bath

7:30 AM: Breakfast

8:00 AM: Mom arrived

8:30 AM: Off to physical therapy to work on my limbs

9:00 AM: Off to speech therapy

10:00 AM: Physio on my arms in the pool

10:30 AM: The baths where the dead skin was scrubbed off my body

11:00 AM: Taken back to my room to sleep until lunch

12:00 PM: Lunch

1:00 PM: Nap

2:00 PM: Awake

3:15 PM: Mom would leave

3:30 PM: Off to occupational therapy

5:00 PM: Supper

5:00-ish PM: Gladys would arrive

6:00 PM: Gladys would leave

6:00–6:15 PM: Dad would arrive

7:30 PM: Dad would leave.

Then I'd fall asleep later until morning.

These times are not exact, and my mom did spend a lot of time visiting me.

The physio on my legs was at times very painful, especially after a skin graft. They would have me straighten my legs all the way. The area on my leg where the skin had been taken hurt when I did this. It was very painful. Because of this, I always tried to hold back a bit, and the physical therapists were constantly scolding me for doing so.

In the Royal Alex, there were curbs along the hallway walls about four to five inches high. I would often walk with my sore leg on the curb so that it would be a little higher off the ground than my other leg, meaning I wouldn't have to straighten it. When the nurses caught me doing this, they told me to stop. I did, but as soon as they left I would start again.

During my entire time in the hospital, I wanted my mom and dad to hold me, to make me feel safe and warm, but I never quite felt like I got the comfort I craved. Part of the reason was that my family didn't want to get my burns infected by getting too close to me. Human contact was not a good plan since I was still so sick, weak, and could catch anything from anyone. The other reason was that I wanted to be held twenty-four hours a day, but that was just not possible.

Once I was healthier and doing better, my mom or dad didn't visit me as often as they had. I spent a lot of time recuperating in bed, straining my ears, hoping to hear someone was coming down the hall to see me. Mom was a soft patter, Dad a heavier tread. Grandma had heels that clicked down the hall. I learned to recognize the sound of the family's footsteps. After I met Gladys, she continued to visit me, even after her son was released. I learned the sound of her footsteps as well as her heels going clickity-click down the hall. Mixed with the cadence and speed of their steps, I could tell them all apart.

Gladys would occasionally surprise me with presents. I recall her bringing a number of blow-up animals of various sizes, one of which was a tiger; I thought they were all fantastic. One day, she brought a new package. I opened it up with excitement and found a deflated animal of some sort inside. Gladys blew it up. It was a deer. It was very tall and came up to my chest when I was standing. I couldn't believe how huge it was; I was delighted. Gladys seemed to love seeing me so happy.

Gladys gave me a hard time sometimes when I was cranky, for not trying hard and for expecting others to compensate for me because of my hardship. She would get right on my case when that happened. On numerous occasions, I'd be lying on my back and my head would be sunk so far into my pillow that it would prevent me from clearly hearing what Gladys was saying to me. On one such occasion, I woke up to see Gladys in my room. When she saw that I was awake, she came to my bedside and leaned over and started talking to me, but the pillow prevented me from fully hearing her, especially if I was lying on my side.

"What?" I said after the third time. I was getting a little exasperated, not being able to hear her. A few minutes went by with me saying "What?" to every question, because the pillow muffled the sound of her voice.

One day, Gladys got mad at me and told me that if I couldn't quite hear what others were saying I should try reading their lips. At least that's how I recall it; it's funny how we remember things. When corresponding with Gladys about it years later, she recalled it differently: "I don't remember talking harshly to you. I never would have done that. Gosh, you were in so much pain and I had so much respect and admiration and love for that little boy who was valiantly struggling for his life. You were a HERO in my eyes."

CHAPTER 12

....

LIES!

Dave, Age 6

As a young boy, I may have translated Gladys' suggestion that I learn to lip-read as her getting upset at me. Regardless, I gave it a try and once Gladys saw that I was trying, she helped me along by speaking more slowly. I became quite good at reading lips after that, but only when I could partially hear the person. Watching their lips helped me to fill in the blanks.

I looked forward to Gladys' visits as much as my family's, and I would even get upset occasionally when she was late.

One day she came twenty minutes late. For me, it seemed an eternity. I was getting madder by the minute, and when she finally came into the room all harried from trying to get to my room as quickly as she could, I poured out all the emotion that had been building up.

I shouted at her as loud as I could.

"You're late!" I screamed. "And you're wearing black! *I hate black!*"

Gladys seemed to understand that I had spoken those words out of my loneliness and emotion welling up in me. I often felt abandoned when one of my visitors didn't show up on time. Because she was late, I was feeling as if she might not come at all, and so I lashed out. She seemed to understand that and never held it against me.

She often helped me with things I couldn't do on my own, and one area where she was particularly helpful was when my skin grafts started to itch as they healed up. The areas on my arms and back were the worst. I would nearly be going mad from the itching when Gladys would arrive and apply a special cream, gently rubbing it in to stop the itching.

I celebrated my sixth birthday in the Glenrose Hospital. By then, I was up and around much more and was allowed to watch television. I was mesmerized by a regularly-aired commercial advertising a six-wheeled motorized vehicle that could actually drive across small ponds. It was the most fascinating thing to me and I wanted one!

When my birthday arrived, Mom and Dad brought in my present. It was a large box: I just knew it was the vehicle from the commercial. I eagerly opened up the box discovering an orange plastic contraption inside. It had wheels, so that was a good sign, but the vehicle in the commercial wasn't orange, it was green! I felt a bit disappointed.

It only needed the wheels, steering wheel, and horn put on, and my dad had this completed in no time. Once put together it looked just like a tricycle with one wheel in the front and two in the back. The wheels in the back were thick, making it look more like a tractor. Well, it might not have been what I saw on TV but it looked fun and I was no longer disappointed in it. I jumped on it and tore off down the hall, causing a few nurses to jump out of the way.

There was a circuit around the ward so that I never had to turn around; I could just drive around and around the circuit. I would fly down the hall, pedaling like mad and honking my horn. I'd fly around the corner so fast the hard plastic wheels slid along the smooth floor.

I spent a lot of my free time riding my new toy and it was good exercise for me, having spent the majority of the last nine months in bed. No one had to coax me to spend time on it; it was all they could do to hold me back from riding around the halls every waking hour. It was a great motivator. I was more inclined to try harder in all my physio sessions so that I could get back to riding my tractor sooner.

Physical therapy involved repetitive exercise of my limbs. Occupational therapy was similar, but used fun activities that got me moving my limbs. If anyone in the hospital had put me on the tractor, it would have been the occupational therapy department.

Mom would come to visit me sometimes only to find I was not in my room. She'd ask the nurses where I was.

"Oh he's on his tractor," one of them would reply with a smile.

Then she'd see me come screeching around the corner, heading straight to meet her.

My mom has said she can still picture me pedaling as fast as I could so that the tractor drifted around the corner, my hospital gown billowing out behind me.

I spent a lot of time in therapy not only to learn how to use my hands again but to strengthen my legs, test my hearing, and learn how to speak properly. Some of my upper lip had been melted off in the fire and I couldn't close my mouth completely. Though the doctors had plans to fix my mouth, the plans were not immediate and as it turned out they never did get around to it. So I had to learn to talk without the use of my lips, and this was a long, frustrating road.

I had a good speech therapist who would show me the position of her tongue in her mouth as she pronounced different letters. Some letters were easy, but the really hard ones for me to master were P, B, M, N, V, F and WH sounds. Some of these are the sounds we form by touching our lips together, and for me that was no longer an option.

My hearing was also tested, since my outer ears, earflaps, and lobes had been burned off and the doctors wanted to find out if there had been any internal damage. The main purpose of the outer ear is to capture sound and funnel it to the inner ear. The plastic surgeon tried to construct earflaps for me a few times using skin and cartilage from elsewhere on my body, but they never lasted.

The testing, however, was positive and I had no hearing loss. I did have a hard time sometimes determining which direction a sound came from, not in the controlled sound booth at the Glenrose but out on the street, with the wind and street sounds throwing me off. I didn't seem to have any more difficulty in this than anyone else, though. I didn't seem to miss my outer ears except later in life when I wished I had them to hang my sunglasses on!

The Glenrose School had Grades One through Twelve. I had missed starting Grade One back in September, and since it was so late in the school year and those in charge didn't want to overtax me, they placed me in kindergarten from March through June. I only went until noon each day and I didn't go every day due to my surgery schedules. When I did go, I fell asleep a lot because I tired quickly. The cartoons and kids' shows put me to sleep and I often woke up back in bed.

I'm sure I used all the spare energy I had at this point riding my new tractor—that is, if I had any left over after physical and occupational therapy.

It was hard for me at the Glenrose, since I spent more time awake, which meant more time alone without visitors. When my mom came to visit, I so longed for her company that when it was time for her to leave I was heartbroken. I ached for her to stay. I still missed my grandma's visits, which made my mom's departures tougher.

Thankfully, this did not happen every day because Gladys came to visit a lot and planned her visits to coincide just after Mom left. She could not make it every day, though, and I have haunting memories of being left behind while my mom hurried to catch the bus before Keir arrived home from school.

Most of the nurses were understanding, but this did not make it any easier for me. I would follow my mom to the stairwell and call for her to come back. I'd tell her

I had one more thing I had to say. She would stop on her way down the stairs, several flights down by then, and call out for me to tell her what it was. But I had nothing to say, I had only the empty ache in my heart that said, "Don't leave me! I don't want to be alone!"

Most of the nurses would try to convince me to leave the stairwell, but they were never successful until I heard the door at the bottom of the stairs slam shut and I knew for certain that Mom was gone.

One night, one of the nurses thought it best to remove me from the situation when my mom started down the stairs and I began my routine. I'm sure she thought it would be easier for me. She pulled me away from the railing, out of the stairwell, and down the hall to my room. Then, being kind, she knelt down in front of me to try and ease the pain I was feeling. But I was hopping mad!

I kicked her right smack in the chest. She took off all my clothes as punishment so I wouldn't run out of my room, then put me to bed. I fell asleep that night with that now-familiar dull, empty ache which I couldn't seem to shake.

In the spring, the hospital held events for the Cub Scouts (for the boys) and Brownies, which is part of the Girl Guides (for the girls). I planned to join the Cub Scouts, but when the doctors heard there were some Cub activities that took place outside, they sent word that I would not be allowed to join. They were not going to take any chances with my health since the weather was not very warm yet.

I was devastated and my roommate at the time wouldn't stop talking about how excited he was to be in the Cub Scouts. I couldn't really blame him, but I wished he'd rant about it somewhere else.

I was incredibly crushed that I would not be allowed to take part in the Cubs. A few days later, I was told that I might be permitted, as a special consideration, to join the Brownies. I thought that was ridiculous! Surely the girls did nothing in their meetings that would excite a boy.

As it turned out, the Brownies hung out once a week and had lots of snacks to eat. I decided to join and helped them polish off those snacks. The meetings took place in the evenings and I was usually out of energy by then. The girls were awesome and would make me comfortable, bringing me something to eat and drink. I was such a novelty to them that one or more of the girls were constantly coming over to see if I needed anything.

There weren't any comfy chairs that I recall, so I usually ended up lying on the floor on top of the girls' jackets. As the evening progressed and some of the girls got tired, a few of them would come and snuggle up on the pile of jackets. As a six-year-old, I couldn't think of anything more blissful than the Brownies meetings. I didn't really participate in any activities with the girls, so I have no recollection what they did in their meetings. I almost always fell asleep before the end, waking up the next morning in my bed.

The month of June arrived, marking my one-year anniversary in the hospital. Mom told the doctors that she knew everything I needed done for my health and that she was taking me home to live. This was not a request; this was a statement. And I went home. I cannot describe the peace that flooded my heart knowing that as I went to bed each night, my mom was nearby if I needed her for anything.

I would still be sent back to the hospital for more surgeries, but except for post-surgery recuperation I would live at home. I was sent back to the Royal Alex later that very summer for more work. While I was recuperating, the nurses introduced me to the games room on the second floor where I was staying.

There was an enormous pool table in the games room. The funny thing about it was that there was no cue ball. Maybe it was left out of the game on purpose to make it easier for kids. I got quite good at playing and beat the nurses regularly, though I'm sure ninety-nine percent of the time it was because they let me win. This winning was a good morale booster for me.

A month or two later, I was back in the hospital for more surgery. While I was there, Grandma came back to Edmonton to visit us. She was quite shocked by the appearance of both Keir and I, who had just recently undergone more treatment. She hadn't seen us for several months and wasn't used to our altered appearances. Keir recently had work done on his mouth while I'd had work done on my hands, head, and eyelids. She described me in a letter to her sister:

> He looks like a little creature with a mask…but he seems happy and full of chuckles. Roberta said that when she felt despondent, she would go see Dave and it would cheer her up. He is so confident, self-reliant, and happy.

She finished her thoughts with this: "Keir and Dave are both happy and busy and interested in life. Can I be less?"

*   *   *

In the fall, I was back in the Glenrose as a student, while still living at home. I was starting Grade One a year later than I should have because of the fire, but at least I was there now. I rode the school bus to and from school. I was picked up right at the door of my house and driven to the school entrance and back. I often slept both ways.

In fact, when the bus pulled up at my house to drop me off, my mom often had to go out to the bus and carry me, still sleeping, into the house.

At school, I became the class clown, perhaps in an effort to help deal with my difficulties and new adjustments; I was kicked out of class numerous times for cracking jokes.

I wish I could remember more incidents, but I only remember one. I was up out of my desk one day, as usual. I was known to help several of the students with math, some of those kids with mental difficulties. I did this often with the permission of the teacher since I found the math easy. But on this particular day, the teacher told me to get back in my desk. Instead, trying to get a few laughs, I tried to fit my legs under the writing surface where my pencils and notebooks were stored.

The teacher was not amused and sent me out in the hall. This was not the first time I'd ended up there. I slouched in the corner by the door, but as usual I didn't have to stay there long: I was usually whisked away within a short time for physical therapy, speech therapy, or to have my hearing tested.

I enjoyed school for the most part, but there were some people who made my time there unpleasant. One particular boy and his sister made my life miserable by following me around all the time. When they caught me alone, they ridiculed me.

"Our mom says you got burned playing with fire."

That's a lie! my mind screamed.

I told them it wasn't true.

"My mom says it is!" the boy would say. "She says you deserve what you got for playing with fire…"

CHAPTER 13

....

PUBLIC SCHOOL

Dave, Ages 6½–9

I had never played with fire, but these two kids weren't there to ask me what happened. They were there to tell me. To tell me what their mom had told them—that I deserved what I got.

I wanted to cry. How could I fight their mother's lies when she wasn't even there? I was only six years old and didn't know how to fight this lie, so I avoided them as much as I could.

Another boy also took a dislike to me, and one time when I was walking down a deserted hall at school he came through the double doors in the center of the hallway

126   DAVE HAMMER

and tried to scratch my eyes. He got me with his fingernail and just walked away. When I put my hand to my eyes I looked down to see blood.

I stumbled off to the nursing station. The nurse laid me down on the little cot to look at my eye. Thankfully, the boy hadn't scratched my actual eye; he'd only scratched the skin by the corner of my eye. During the examination, the sight of my own blood was too much for me and I passed out.

When I came to, the nurse was peering anxiously into my face. Other than feeling a bit unsteady on my feet, I was just fine. I kept a tissue applied to the corner of my eye until the bleeding stopped.

I was still being sent back to the Royal Alex for operations. At one point, I was moved up to the third floor of the Royal Alex where there was rumored to be a very mean nurse. I had many skin grafts taken from my legs and applied to my upper body. Once my leg had healed enough, the nurses would remove the dressing. Most of them let me soak it off in the bathtub. In later years, that method proved unsanitary, and instead a little bit of saline solution was used. In my case, the tub was used or it was peeled off dry.

The first encounter with the Mean Nurse was shortly after my next skin graft. I had a dressing on the back of my thigh and she had me stand on a chair, then insisted on peeling off the dressing right then and there. I begged and pleaded for the bandage to be soaked off and finally she agreed.

Happily, I turned to step off the chair, but just as I did the nurse caught hold of the dressing and tore it off in one fluid motion. The hot pain shot up my leg and through my entire body. My screams echoed through the halls. She had lied to me.

Even though most of the nurses and other health care workers went out of their way to help me feel at home, this one nurse killed my trust for all the rest. Afterwards, my mistrust of nurses grew. I didn't turn my back on them again.

Despite this, I still had a good time with a lot of the nurses. Some would come to my room on their break to see if there was anything I wanted before they headed off to the nearby store.

A favorite game of mine involved practicing my hand-eye coordination. The nurses would set up an empty bucket across the room by the door and I would practice tossing my crayons into it. When I ran out of crayons, I'd buzz the nurses. One of them would come to collect all the crayons and put them back on my lap so I could start again. I was a pretty good shot by the time I walked out of the hospital for the last time.

The nurses never *seemed* to tire of collecting my crayons when I played this game, although I'm sure they probably did. I was a good-natured boy who had been through a terrible ordeal so the majority of the nurses, with their kind hearts were glad to do almost anything for me. On occasion, they would even help me color in my coloring book.

One time I had gone for surgery and I was back in the Royal Alex recovering. I spent a few hours painting with watercolors, rinsing my brush in a glass of water whenever I switched to a new color. Later, a nurse came in and told me I needed to finish my juice. I had no idea what she was talking about. There was no juice on my little table. Then, to my horror, she picked up my paint water, gesturing for me to drink it. That's when I noticed the water did look a bit like apple juice.

"That's paint water!" I managed to croak.

"Don't give me that! You're just trying to get out of drinking this."

I pointed helplessly to my paintbrush and paints, but she wasn't buying it. Apparently, in her mind, I had staged the paints and paintbrushes to get out of drinking my juice.

She tried to pour the yellowish water into my mouth, but I clamped it shut and refused to cooperate. She might have gotten some of it down my throat if my mom hadn't walked into the room right then.

"What are you doing?" she asked, striding over to the nurse. "That's the water he's been dipping his paintbrush in!"

I saw the look of sudden realization on the nurse's face. She looked chagrined.

*   *   *

Going to school at the Glenrose was easy. I fit right in, because everyone there had some sort of physical or mental difficulty. I remember quite a lot of things about the kids at school, but I do not remember many names. Of the students I do recall, two of them became close friends.

One of these was a girl named Joanne, who was in a wheelchair. I hit it off with Joanne in Grade Two and we became inseparable. With two great senses of humor, we made each other laugh constantly. But it wasn't all laughing;

I wheeled her around in her chair and we explored every inch of the school, every hallway, every nook and cranny. I loved hanging out with Joanne and hearing her laugh.

We lost touch when I left the Glenrose, but I've always remembered her character, awesome sense of humor, and easy laugh. The ease with which we could get along became a rare thing in my life.

Peter was the other good friend I made in the school hospital. We got to know each other on the bus. He had multiple sclerosis (MS) and was confined to a wheelchair. The last few rows of seats on the bus were removed to make room for those in wheelchairs. I sat near the back of the bus, and that's how Peter and I started talking and discovered we lived close to each other in St. Albert. From then on, I always tried to get the last seat in the back of the bus so we could talk. We also started to hang out after school.

Peter did not have much strength in his arms and could not lift them without assistance. One way he got around this was to plant his elbow on his leg, lower his head, grab a hold of his hair with his hand, and hold on while he lifted his head, taking his arm up with it. This way he could get his arm onto a table, a desk, or the arms of his wheelchair.

One of the first times I met Peter, I was pestering him, as young kids will sometimes do, and since he couldn't use his arms to get at me, he waited until my hand was close and then struck. He clamped my hand in his mouth, bit down hard, and held on. That straightened me out in a hurry, and I had to use my wits to convince him to let go. He got me more than once and it sure hurt. I could see his teeth marks in my hand!

Another student, named Claire, seemed smart enough to me, but she lacked confidence in herself. She had a musculature disease that didn't allow her to control her muscles very well. I often worked with her. She had a pointer board she used to communicate. The board had the letters of the alphabet and certain commonly used words she could point to, to spell a word or complete a phrase. Claire could speak, but it was very garbled and hard to understand. Her mouth muscles were distorted and didn't work properly, garbling her speech and causing her to drool. I could tell she was terribly embarrassed about this.

I spent time helping her, because most of the other kids couldn't understand or relate to her. I couldn't really, either, at least not right away. But after a while I could understand her speech bit by bit and saw that beneath this debilitating disease Claire had feelings and needs and was a person just as much as I was.

It seemed to me that once I was at ease with Claire and she realized it, her movements became less jerky, and this calmness allowed her muscles to operate a bit more smoothly.

Part of my daily occupational therapy involved taking a baking class where I learned to make cakes. I sifted flour, added the ingredients, and mixed it all together. It was fun. Once the cake was cooked, we performed my favorite part: mixing up the icing and adding a little food coloring to make the icing whatever color I liked. Green, pink, blue, and yellow; these were some of the colors I chose. I loved bright colors.

Once the icing was applied and everything was complete, the occupational therapist wrapped the cake in plastic wrap, but not before putting toothpicks on top to keep the plastic off the icing. It was always exciting to bring home my latest cake and show off the icing color. Mom was always excited to see my latest creation.

All the hair on my head had been burned off in the fire and the roots were so badly damaged that no hair would grow except for one spot at the base of my neck. It must have been protected by my pillow at the time of the fire. That area was burned less severely and it delighted me that hair did grow there.

The doctors thought I might be better accepted for my appearance if they could fashion a wig for me. They ordered one, matching the hair I already had. I wore it for a while, but as my head grew it fit less well. Then one day in the school coatroom I had a disagreement with another boy who tried to pull my hair, not knowing I wore a wig. It came off right in his hand and I felt humiliated. After that, I started wearing the wig less and less.

Every Easter, the Glenrose put on a tea where they served strawberry shortcake. It wasn't until I had been there a year or two that I was healthy enough to attend. My mom came and I got all dressed up. Sitting at the table with all the adults was so exciting for me that I got very animated with wild gesturing, telling my mom about some of my recent accomplishments. I knocked my drink over, dousing the poor lady beside me. She was quick to tell me it was okay, but I was already embarrassed. I was quiet the rest of the meal, but at the end of it all I really did have an enjoyable time.

By the end of Grade Three, I was much better at using my hands. I could print quite well (using both my hands to hold the pencil) and pick things up more easily. I got to ride a big three-wheeled bicycle up and down the halls of the school, which I loved. I could feed myself without any straps simply from hours of practice. I could also dress myself without the use of any aids. My shirts had Velcro instead of buttons, since I hadn't reached the stage where I was ready to try buttons yet. This would come later.

I attended three years in the children's hospital school, and over that time I heard many unpleasant stories about the fourth-grade teacher, Mrs. Pritchard. I was terrified of getting to Grade Four and being in her class, but as it would turn out I had nothing to worry about.

When I finished Grade Three, word came that I would not be attending the Glenrose School the following year but would instead be placed in the St. Albert public school system. It was such a relief not to be put in Grade Four at the children's hospital. Instead I would be heading to a new place. I felt an air of excitement.

The summer went by quickly and I spent most of my time reading, which had become a passion of mine. In fact, I would take out so many books at a time that the Glenrose put a limit on how many I could check out at once. I was taking out about forty books at a time and keeping them for two weeks, seriously depleting their rather small stock. The new limit was twenty, but that didn't slow me down. I simply took out twenty, returned them in a week, and took out twenty more.

When I wasn't reading, I was over at Peter's house playing with him and his toys, or hanging out in the backyard with him and his dad. Peter's dad kept St. Bernard dogs, two of which were always in the annual summer parade.

As a young boy, I was awestruck at the size of these dogs, and I even got to ride on their backs a few times.

When my dad had time off that summer, a year after the fire, he took us all to Jasper National Park. Even though I was still quite weak, I was able to do many of the things I wanted to. Afterward, I was always exhausted. We went on an all-uphill hike and my parents kept expecting me to tire out, but I made it all the way to the top of the lookout.

While in the mountains, my parents wanted to have a family service for my sister. My parents had had her body cremated and my mom wanted a family-only memorial service. We rented a canoe and paddled out to the middle of one of the lakes in Jasper and spread her ashes in the water. It was a very sad moment for me at the age of six.

I no longer asked my mom where Kimberly was, for she broke into tears each and every time, making me feel bad that I had asked. I understood that my sister was no longer alive, but that was about the extent of it. My heart ached for her. I missed her dearly. She was never far from my thoughts, and even though I'd been told she was gone I couldn't help expecting to see her at any time, everywhere we went.

Kimberly always used to come to my rescue when Keir playfully beat me up. He'd have me pinned to the carpet hollering, and Kimberly would come running. My sister had a good heart, and I'll always remember her as soft and compassionate.

Back home, after our Jasper trip, the summer was almost over. The fall loomed closer and I looked forward to going to my new school, not knowing the hardships that lay ahead for me.

I wasn't aware of it, but in August, just weeks before the school year started, the principal of the public school I was soon to be attending phoned my mom and asked her to meet him at his office. My mom later told me he wanted to make one thing, and one thing only, perfectly clear, and it was not that he and the school would do everything in their power to make my transition as easy and painless as possible.

Rather, he sat my mom down and, looking her in the eyes, stated in a stern voice, "There will be *no exceptions* and *no allowances* made here for your son."

CHAPTER 14

....

KISS ME

Dave, Ages 9–11

My mother was speechless. I didn't need much in the way of exceptions or allowances, but it would have been nice if they had offered. The only help I really needed was to be in the front row so I could read the blackboard. My tear ducts had been damaged beyond repair in the fire, so my eyes often welled up with tears blurring my vision. They had gotten better with time, but in Grade Four it was still a problem.

Despite the principal's words, my mom didn't breathe a word of it to me until many years later.

On the first day of school, I headed off with excitement mixed with a bit of apprehension. The schoolyard was just across the back alley from us, so I only had to scale the schoolyard fence and walk across the grass to the school. Around the side of the building were two sets of double doors. I was a bit nervous pushing through them for the first time. I didn't know anyone at this school, and that made me a bit apprehensive, but I expected I would be accepted just as I had been at the Glenrose.

At the Glenrose, everyone had some sort of obvious difference, but here in this new school it was apparent that I was the only one with readily identifiable differences. When I stood in a group, all eyes picked me out of the crowd. The Sesame Street song "Which of these things is not like the others, which of these things just doesn't belong?" felt like it was written just for me. I didn't feel different from the other children, but I knew I stood out.

I always got reactions when I went out in public. Public school was no different; some thought I looked like a freak, others were fearful around me, and still others found my appearance repulsive.

Yet how was that my fault? Was it my fault that while I slept at age five a fire started in the tent and burned around me leaving me so badly burned that all my fingers were amputated and my face was left a permanent scar? I knew firmly in my heart that it wasn't, and I did my best not to let the reactions of others deter me in any way.

Somehow the girls were different. Most of them took to me right away. I often found myself surrounded by them at recess.

"What happened? Do your hands hurt when you touch things?" April would ask in her sweet young voice.

"Not anymore," I'd say.

"Do you need a lot of help doing things?"

They had a lot of questions and I never grew tired of answering them. It wasn't often that I got this much attention and concern from my peers.

The girls liked touching my skin because it felt different and it intrigued them. I had outgrown my wig, so I was baldheaded. They touched me on my arms, neck, face, and head. When they found out that I didn't have feeling on all parts of my scalp due to the severity of the burns, the girls enjoyed touching me on all different parts of it to see whether I could feel it or not.

"Can you feel this?" Susan would ask.

"How about this?" Tina piped up, moving her fingers quickly from one spot to the next.

I responded anytime I could actually feel the touch, but with so many people touching my head at once, their fingers dancing lightly over my skin, they often passed the spot by the time I could answer them. Then they'd take the time to hunt that spot back down.

Not everyone took to me like these girls did, but it would take me a while to find that out.

Being bald at school was okay, but one day while walking home I found a baseball cap and decided to bring it home to wash and wear. From that time on, I wore a baseball cap every day. The nice thing about the cap was that it shielded my eyes from the sun. My eyes, because of the severity of the burns, were no longer able to close, so it was a welcome relief to have some shade.

The classrooms in public school were run differently from the Glenrose. At the Glenrose, there were often students out of their chairs helping other students because so many had physical or mental difficulties to overcome. There, students were asked by the teacher to help out during math, science, and spelling exercises. At public school, everyone remained in their seats unless called out by the teacher. It was simply a matter of getting used to a slightly different system, which was okay by me. It seemed easy enough.

I took to everything in the new school, including sports and gym, which I'd had limited exposure to at the Glenrose. In gym, there was one act of strength that all the kids practiced called the flexed-arm hang, which was similar to a chin-up. This was where you held onto a bar with both hands and pulled yourself up until your chin lifted above the bar while your feet dangled below. The object was to hold oneself there as long as possible. As soon as your chin dipped below the bar, time was stopped. The gym teacher put all the students into a competition to see who could hang for the longest.

I loved participating in all the sports at school, but at first I didn't participate in this event because I couldn't grip the bar with my hands. After watching all the other kids take turn after turn, day after day, I devised a plan for how I could also hang up there. This really appealed to my competitive nature. I ran it by the gym teacher, who spent a couple days considering it and decided my technique would be acceptable.

At the next gym class, I climbed up to the bar, hanging by the crooks of my arms. I put my forearms over the bar, pulled myself upwards with my upper arm and shoulder muscles, and proceeded to hang that way for two minutes, almost a full minute longer than the other boys. The class watched in amazement. I felt great. One lad declared my method unfair and easy. I let him try. He lasted five seconds before dropping to the floor.

"That hurts!" he hollered as he ran out of the gymnasium.

I had to agree with him.

*   *   *

I read a lot in my free time, partly because I didn't have a lot of friends, but in time that would change.

My homeroom teacher, Mr. Ginsett, was my English teacher, and Mrs. Caruthers taught social studies. My most vivid memory of Mrs. Caruthers was the time she had to leave the classroom for a moment and asked Rachel, one of the students, to write "Whisper"' on the blackboard. Then she left.

Rachel sauntered up to the blackboard and wrote "Whisper Pantyhose." The class erupted with laughter. Mrs. Caruthers had a fit when she returned. I'm not sure what punishment Rachel received, but she had won the respect of the class for her gutsiness.

Grade Four went by quickly. I did well in school and continued to excel at the flexed arm hang, setting the mark high for other students to aim for. They eventually caught up to me, turning it into a real competition, which I thrived on.

I always wanted to try new things, so when an older boy showed me how to steal, I was open to it. He taught me how to watch when no one was looking and where to stick the item where it wouldn't be noticed. On my first attempt with a few friends, we all made it out of the store except one, my closest friend, Rodney. He was caught, his parents were called, and he wasn't allowed to hang out with me after that.

He was my one good friend and I regretted that I had let stealing ruin our friendship. Had I been given the choice to stop stealing or stop being friends with Rodney, I would have stopped stealing. However, since there was nothing I could do to redeem the friendship in his parents' eyes, I kept right on stealing, but always by myself after that.

I had a hard time making friends at school, but I saw that people were easily put off by my appearance, which instantly spoke to me about their character. I preferred to befriend people who had the depth to look past my appearance. Rodney had been my only good friend in Grade Four and I didn't have another good friend at school until Grade Five.

My friendship with Sean was a memorable part of the fifth grade. We met in the school playground and became inseparable. After that, we played together during recess and hung out after school, usually at his house, which was just a few doors down from mine. We hung out nonstop that year and I slept over at his house a few times on weekends. I felt like part of his family. On one sleepover, we watched a movie that terrified me, and on advice from his mom I never told my parents. I was sad to see him go when he moved to Kamloops, British Columbia a year later.

During fifth grade, my homeroom teacher announced that there would be a reading competition to see who could read the most books in one month. We were not allowed to count any books we had previously read or any of the thin children's books. The student who read the most pages would win. I was determined from the onset to be the winner.

I wasted no time, starting to read on the first day of the competition and dutifully writing each book down on my list. Within a week and a half, I had read a dozen books. We were required to periodically hand in our book list so the teacher could see our progress. That way, if one of the students had a blank page for the first twenty-eight days of the month, the teacher would know they were cheating if they had twenty books on their list at the end.

The first time I handed in my list, I arrived home to find out that my teacher had called my mom to make sure I was following the rules of the competition.

"Now, you know he can only count books that he's read since the first of March," she told my mom.

"He is," my mom replied.

"Oh, well, then he isn't supposed to be reading thin little books!"

"He's not! All these books are at least a hundred pages long with no pictures in them!"

I was so proud that my mom defended me.

I was so far ahead of the others in the competition that one girl, Rochelle, said she was going to read the dictionary so she'd beat me in pages read. I thought about doing that, too, but it sounded so boring that I just kept reading books from the library. At the end of the month, I had read twice as many books as Rochelle, who placed second.

I had won. As a reward, I received a macramé wall hanging of a frog, which I proudly hung on my wall. It felt so good to win a prize for something.

Near the end of the school year, we went on a school trip where we hiked, swam, and used compasses in the woods. I had a blast!

But greater than friendship, accomplishments, or an awesome school trip was Susan. Susan was a friendly red-head and the first girl that I was aware of who had a crush on me. She pestered and bugged me to no end until one day I wrestled her to the ground and told her I'd kiss her if she didn't stop.

"Kiss me?" she asked with a small smile on her lips.

CHAPTER 15

STUCK-UP BRAT!

Dave, Ages 11–12

Seeing that Susan wanted me to kiss her scared me, so I quickly changed my mind. I often thought later that I should have kissed her, but I was too young—only ten at the time.

As I grew older, I became more independent and would ride my bike to the mall by myself where I continued to steal small items like fishing lures, small squirt guns, and pens. I stole only occasionally until one day I came home with a few items and took them to my room. That's when Mom started calling for me and, when I went to see her, she had a stern look on her face which I hadn't seen before.

She had somehow figured out that I didn't have the money to pay for the things I'd just brought back from the store. After having a serious talk with me, Mom forced me to take the items back. I never stole again after that.

In retrospect, I am very glad she caught on. If she hadn't, I might have kept on stealing until the signs were gone, the signs that warned me it was wrong: sweaty palms, butterflies in the stomach, and the guilt pricking at my conscience. If I'd continued long enough, I would have killed those feelings. I much preferred the ease of mind when I paid for items as opposed to how I felt after shoplifting.

Going into public places was difficult, due to the negative reactions I received from people. As I got older and became more aware, I found that it was very hard to deal with. I started withdrawing emotionally. Home was the only environment where I was treated for who I was and not for what I looked like. School didn't feel like a safe place, and public places were even worse.

The reactions I received were varied, from parents in stores gasping involuntarily when they saw me, to hearing things being whispered when I was by myself. I often heard kids asking their parents why I looked so funny.

"Mom what happened to that guy?"

"Dad, look at that monster over there!"

"That guy is so ugly, I wonder what happened to him…?"

Sometimes kids would simply pull on their parents' clothing to get their attention while gawking at me the whole time.

Out on the street, I got variations of the same thing: "Hey take off your mask! Don't you know Halloween is over?"

In fact, the last time I got a comment like this wasn't long ago and I simply replied, "I'm not. I was in a fire."

One day in a furniture store, a woman, obviously perturbed, asked me, "Why would you wear a mask in here?"

Fed up with that question, I shot back at her, "It's not a mask!"

I had my hands in my pockets the whole time, and as we looked at each other I pulled my left hand out of my pocket to scratch my nose. She took one look at my hands and, looking embarrassed, got up and left. It wasn't until afterwards that I realized she stopped thinking I was wearing a mask only when she saw my burned hands.

All these reactions were terribly unpleasant, so I stopped going out unless I was with friends or family. I began to withdraw, becoming more and more shy. I spent more time at home reading and building new things with Lego, a favorite toy of mine.

Once when I was six, someone very gently advised me that I would probably never be able to ride a bike. This only fuelled my desire to try. I pestered and begged my parents for a bicycle, and that Christmas I received a brand new one from Gladys! Boy, was I excited! It had training wheels so I could hop on it right away and zip round and round the house, completing a circuit that took me through the living room, dining room, kitchen, hall, and back into the living room again. It was so much fun that I didn't want to get off.

As soon as spring arrived, I took my bike outside and rode it for months. When summer came, I asked my dad to take off the training wheels and, after doing so, he taught me to ride solo.

A couple days later, when Dad came home from work, I was despondent, because I couldn't seem to master the art of balancing on the bike. I begged him to put the training wheels back on, but instead he sat me down and told me I could do it; I just had to keep trying.

With the confidence my father instilled in me, I rode my bike the next day, sure that I could balance without the training wheels. After only a couple of runs, I was doing it! I couldn't wait to show Dad when he came home that evening.

I rode that bike for a year or two before outgrowing it. Mom found me a bigger one at a yard sale, and even though it was a little too big, I was determined to master it.

When I first started riding a bike, I grasped the handlebars with the crooks of my arms and leaned right over them. I did this until I hit a big hole in the road once and, because I was so far forward on the bike, I went right over the handlebars and landed on my head.

After this, I taught myself how to hold onto the handlebars a different way, learning to grasp the handlebars with just my hands. I practiced and practiced until I finally mastered it and my bike-riding got even better.

*   *   *

In Grade Six, I started at the Junior High school next door where I didn't know anyone in my homeroom class. In fact, none of my friends had come with me to this new school, so I had to start making friends all over again.

One particular classmate took a dislike to me and I was always looking for some way to get him off my back.

It turned out that the whole grade was placed into four different-colored sports teams for the year, and he and I ended up on the green team. By default we became friends to a certain extent—mostly out of convenience. I'd say things like "Hey, the green team is going to win!" or "Wow, did the green team ever score a lot of points yesterday." I milked that right to the end of school. If we hadn't been teammates, we would have been enemies; I was grateful it was the former.

I got in a couple fights in Grade Six, which I won only because Keir practiced his wrestling moves on me at home. Keir would come home and say, "Here, let me show you this new move." The next thing I'd know, he'd have me on the floor twisted like a pretzel.

I pulled a few of these moves on the kids at school and they were quick to give up. I didn't start these fights, but I often recall finding myself in situations where I was facing another boy while surrounded by a ring of rowdy onlookers.

Soon I had a reputation for being a tough guy. On sports day, when other schools came to ours, some of the visiting toughs heard about me and wanted to have a go at me. Thankfully, no fights erupted and it all came to an end when the biggest kid in the grade took a liking to me. As soon as we began hanging out, no one bothered me again. It was such a relief.

*   *   *

After Christmas that year, my mom and dad started talking about getting back together. They did, and in early

March, seven years after they'd separated, we moved to a new house about half a mile away. Due to the distance, I could no longer sleep in, climb over the fence, and simply run across the schoolyard to class. I didn't mind the walk too much, though, since it meant my parents were back together again and I could see my dad every day. A few years later, I had a new brother and sister. Though I was much older than them, they were a blessing to me over the years.

A short time after we moved, there was an announcement on the school intercom telling us that there would be school dances put on every Wednesday by the social club, for a small fee. The first dance was to take place that very day. Though I had become more and more shy, when I heard this announcement I ran home as fast as I could to get the money to go.

I was too shy to ask anyone to dance, but luckily the girls asked me to dance with them during the slow songs. From then on, I never missed a single dance.

In addition to attending the dances, I took up playing basketball. I learned how to shoot underhand until I was quite good, and then practiced until I could shoot overhand. It took longer for me to do this well, as my hands were not flat and the ball would fly off them at a slightly different angle each time.

Life held a lot of challenges for me, yet I grew to enjoy them. What I didn't enjoy were people who assumed I couldn't do things based solely on my appearance. I set out to make it my ambition to prove them wrong each and every time. They didn't always tell me with words that they thought I couldn't accomplish much; instead they said it with their eyes, and I grew to know those looks.

One of my neighborhood friends was sitting on her front porch one summer day with her boyfriend, watching me shoot a basketball in my driveway. I was beginning to have a decent shot. After watching me for a while, her boyfriend came up to me and asked if I wanted to play twenty-one.

I knew how to play the game: you shot from the free throw line, and each point shot from that line was worth two points except for the first shot to start the game, which was only worth one. After any miss, the opponent shot the ball from wherever it was caught and you had to make your shot from there to get one more point and earn another shot from the free throw line. The first person to get exactly twenty-one points won. If they had nineteen points, got a rebound and made the shot they'd have twenty points. Then they'd have to go to the free throw line and miss so as not to go over twenty-one.

My opponent changed the rules and said all shots were worth one point. That was fine by me, but he was looking at me as if I didn't stand a chance. I found that surprising, because he'd just been watching me make shot after shot.

The way he looked at me made me pretty mad. He told me I could go first, so we picked a starting line on the driveway and I began. This smugness ticked me off enough that I brought my A-game and sank twenty-one shots in a row. Game over. He didn't ask for a rematch. This was the only time in my life that I sank that many shots in a row.

Overall I didn't enjoy sixth grade; I had few friends, was generally left out of groups, and some of the teachers didn't seem to care for me. I stopped caring about school, and it began to show.

During a history exam that year, which I was totally unprepared for, I wrote at the bottom of the exam that if the answers I'd given were not marked correct I'd meet the teacher out in the parking lot after school. The teacher didn't often stand up for herself, and for whatever irrational reason, I didn't really think of the consequences. I had no intention of being around after school, so I left the class and thought nothing more of it—that is, until I found myself waiting in front of the principal's office.

At that point, I wished I could undo what I'd written on the exam. I was given a stern talking to, my mother was called, and I was in trouble again when I got home.

My dislike of school grew one cold winter day while my mind was drifting in class. I faintly overheard my teacher say, "I saw him in the grocery store and called his name, but he walked right by and ignored me. What a stuck-up little brat!"

CHAPTER 16

PRIVATE SCHOOL

Dave, Ages 12–15

I sat at my desk wondering who she was talking about when all of a sudden my teacher called my name and pointed right at *me*.

Then I remembered I'd been out the day before at the nearby shopping mall dressed in a parka, the hood zipped all the way to my nose, making it difficult to hear. It was bitterly cold out, and I'd gone in through the grocery store entrance. Not until I had made my way through the grocery store and into the mall did I unzip my parka. I had no recollection of hearing my name called. I've never been the sort to ignore a person greeting me.

My teacher's words paralyzed me. The words "stuck-up little brat" rang in my ears. The embarrassment in front of my entire class made me want to crawl into a hole and die. I was humiliated beyond words.

I changed my name that year. At birth, I had been given the name Bruce and until the age of twelve I'd gone by it. I had a hard time pronouncing it because of my burns, though, so in the spring of my twelfth year I chose to switch to my middle name: Dave. It took awhile for everyone, including my parents, to get used to it, but I stuck to it and when I became an adult I legally changed it.[3]

*   *   *

When I first learned to write, the results were little more than chicken scratches. But at least I could read my own writing, as long as it was just written and still fresh in my mind. If some time passed, however, I would often have a hard time reading it.

I grew tired of struggling to decipher my writing and determined to master my penmanship. I worked hard at it. In less than a year, people began commenting on how my writing had become neater than theirs! They were amazed that I could write so neatly because of my hands. The truth was, it had nothing to do with my hands, but rather how hard I tried.

At the age of ten, I was befriended by a woman who lived nearby and talked to me over the fence as I played in my yard. After we got to know each other a bit, she invited me to church and Keir and Mom came along.

---

3   I have referred to myself as "Dave" through the book to make things less confusing for you, the reader.

We started going to church regularly, and it was here that I heard that Jesus loved me. That didn't mean much to me, since I didn't know Jesus. You may as well have told me that the President of the United States loved me. I would have asked, "Why?"

My mom went to the main service and Keir and I went to Sunday school in the basement. My Sunday school teacher sat me down one day after class and wanted to know if I'd like to accept Jesus as my personal savior. All I knew was that I felt an inner warmth at church, so I said yes. I really didn't know what it all meant, but the next day at school I felt clean, like I'd taken a good long hot bath. I was eleven.

By the end of Grade Six, I was starting to hate school. I didn't feel comfortable there at all. I was getting sick more often and my grades, once high, were now barely above passing. I was on a downward slide. Seeing my hardship, my parents moved me into a private school in Grade Seven.

The private school didn't do much to improve things at first, but as the year went on I gradually started gaining more confidence. I went from a D average in Grade Six to a C average by the end of Grade Seven. Grade Eight saw a total transformation in my grades, shooting up to an A average.

I was a stubborn lad, which undoubtedly helped me cling to life after the fire, and to overcome so much. This stubbornness began to show itself in Grade Eight as I circumvented the rules and purposely went right to the edge of the line on rules that didn't make sense or were useless, in my opinion.

The private school had no school bus system and, since I walked to school, I would hang out with my buddies until their parents arrived. Boys will be boys and horse around, so those in charge felt they needed to put a stop to it. My hanging with my friends wasn't getting anybody into trouble. We weren't being destructive or breaking any laws. We might have tussled a bit, but it was never serious. We were simply having fun, the way boys do.

To stop us from tussling, the administration made a rule that once class was over, if you were not waiting for a ride home, you had to leave the grounds immediately. Those waiting were required to stay inside until their parents arrived.

I would leave school, at least as far as the public sidewalk. From there, I would talk to my friends as they came out to get in their parents' cars.

When the administration found out about this, I was hauled into the office where I calmly explained that I had followed the rules and regulations and left school property. Once I was on the sidewalk, I explained, I was on city property and no longer subject to school rules. They didn't look very pleased as I explained this, but I didn't appreciate having to follow rules that were obviously an attempt to stop my friends and I from hanging out after school. We were good kids doing nothing wrong.

After this, the administration changed the rule again to say that if my friends' parents had not yet arrived, I was to leave school. If the parents had arrived, I was to stay at my desk until they had left. My struggle with the school authorities had just begun.

Another thing, which not only showed my stubbornness but also my creativity, was doing my best to avoid going outside during lunch hour in the dead of winter. After eating, it was mandatory to spend the rest of the lunch hour in the schoolyard, regardless of the weather. There was no good reason for this, from my point of view, so I set out to avoid it. When it dawned on me that detentions were to be served at lunch hour inside, I knew I had the solution. I promptly began getting daily detentions.

Four of my friends in this grade got jealous after a while and started doing the same thing. My plan worked for a while, but one day during detention the principal looked up from his desk and saw that the boys filling the row of detention chairs were the same ones who'd been there all week. He put two and two together and soon detentions were to be served after school. I never got another detention after that.

I slowly started using my stubbornness to motivate myself to greater heights and not to fight the administration or anyone else. My strong will was essential in helping me accomplish seemingly insurmountable things, because I would never give up. I learned to manage it, especially when working alongside and getting along with other people.

I was rather bored when I found my way outside during lunch hour, so a few of us started walking to a private field nearby and playing soccer, thanks to the gracious permission of the owners. We played a lot of soccer. I developed strong friendships in Junior High with two brothers, Lindsay and Carlin, and used to go over to their house to play soccer. Later on in college, my friend Tim and I would take on a group of kids at soccer, usually around the age of twelve. It was just the two of us and we preferred to have at least a half-dozen to play against. We beat them handily almost every time, even with our net empty. We trusted that one of us could make it back in time to guard the net if we needed to. Usually there was no need. My Junior High soccer practices would train me well for those future college years.

I took up playing chess with Carlin on our breaks and free periods at school. My brother Keir had taught me how to play a couple years previously, so I knew the basics. I beat Carlin time after time, but he started getting better and would beat me, eventually forcing me to expand my repertoire of moves so I could return the favor. In this way, we both got much better.

Once my academic marks took off, I never looked back. There was always the Honor Roll, which gave me a higher bar to strive for.

Around the age of fourteen, I became more and more interested in girls. One particular girl, Kelly, took the city bus to school and I started walking her to the bus stop after school. It was on my walk home, so it seemed a natural thing to do. I liked her a lot and, in my clumsy sort of way, asked her out in various and sundry ways.

"When pigs fly!" was her response. And from then on, her response remained unvaried. Still, she didn't say it harshly, simply in a perfect way that fit her sense of humor. So I continued to ask and always received this, to me, rather lovely response, yet not the response I ultimately hoped for.

With other girls, I received responses that were rather painful in delivery. One day while standing by Jackie and

Tammy, Jackie turned to Tammy and said with a smile, "You should go out with Dave!"

"Are you serious?"

"Yah, come on. He's a great guy."

"No way, he's ugly!"

I could do without hearing things like that.

I was a burn victim, but I never saw myself different from anyone else. I saw things differently than others, though. For example, I hated it when a few people would gang up on one person. It didn't matter to me whether it was for fun or not, they were still making the person do something they didn't want to do. Perhaps the reason this bothered me so much was because in the hospital, when I was uncooperative with nurses for fear of what they wanted to do to me, a bunch of them would hold me down and force me to cooperate.

When I was fifteen, I was still getting sick more than others my age. I woke up one morning that year with my mouth filled with little bumps or blisters. Within hours, all the little bumps had popped and the inside of my mouth was a raw torture chamber. My mom took me to the doctor and, not being sure what he was dealing with, the doc had me admitted to the hospital.

I had a specialist look at me because a few similar cases had shown up. The sores healed up by themselves, but through the testing that was performed they found out that I also had pneumonia. That was the second case of pneumonia I'd contracted.

*   *   *

At the end of my fifteenth summer, our household shrunk when Keir left for college. That's when I wanted to leave home, too, especially when we found out that there was a private high school on the same college campus that used the same type of curriculum as my current school.

I wanted to go badly, because I liked the idea of going to school where Keir was. But when my dad heard the cost, he said there was no way he was going to pay for it, and the subject was closed.

CHAPTER 17

....

BOARDING SCHOOL

Dave, Ages 15–16

My dad had a light side and enjoyed playing practical jokes on us kids. When I was three, Kimberly, Keir, and I were sitting on the kitchen counter watching Dad make sandwiches. As he buttered the bread, he unexpectedly reached over and buttered each of our noses. He laughed uproariously at the sight of us: three stunned youngsters with a dash of butter on each nose.

Supper times were another time when Dad liked to play jokes. If any one of us kids got up to get something during the meal, we often returned to find our plate missing. Dad would have snagged it and placed it on his lap, out of sight beneath the table or unseen on an empty chair. As soon as we discovered where it was, he'd hand it over. It usually went like this:

"Dad where's my plate?"

Dad smiling broadly, "I don't know."

"Dad! You have it on your lap!"

Laughingly, "No, I don't."

Then he'd hand it off to another family member or slide it onto an empty chair. Once this was done, he'd slide his chair back and show us he didn't have it. Eventually, through persistence, the plate would be located.

Dad had a lot of fun playing these jokes. He enjoyed being part of our lives, and this seemed to be his way of joining in.

When Dad was six, his father passed away. His mother didn't remarry until his teens, so he didn't have a male role model during those years. This had a big impact on him, but my dad tried to be a good father the best way he knew how.

Some of my favorite times were with Dad on camping trips when we visited his family in Washington State, or my mom's family down in Oregon.

On some family vacations, we'd head for the mountains and Dad would challenge me to footraces. The older I got, the harder he pushed himself to beat me. I'd be sprinting down the gravel road in the campground, my legs pumping as fast as they could and, if I started to pass Dad, he would start laughing and then run even faster and pass me for the win. He made competition fun this way. I couldn't beat him in a footrace until I was fourteen.

Dad was a long distance runner, and he sometimes signed Keir and me up to run cross-country races with him. I never really trained for running, so I usually came across the finish line in the middle of the pack. It wasn't that I was a great runner and didn't need training, but I always pushed myself hard, otherwise I would have quit halfway through the race when my chest was heaving and I couldn't get enough air into my lungs.

Christmastime was when I saw Dad's sense of fun the most. He had a unique way of wrapping presents and hiding them. It was not uncommon to open a present from Dad only to find a can of food or an old book with a note directing us towards the real gift, expertly hidden. The directions were not always clear, often just a clue. When Dad was feeling particularly creative, one note would lead to another present containing another note, and sometimes on and on it would go.

One time, Dad filled a huge box with cans, weights, and other paraphernalia, wrapped it up and addressed it to Mom. Inside, amongst all the cans and weights, my mom found another wrapped present, but it was addressed to Evan, my younger brother.

Christmas was always full of surprises, and through Dad's example we all learned to use creativity and cleverness in our gift-wrapping.

*   *   *

Early in the summer, a year after Keir had gone away to college, something happened to make it possible for me to go away to school with Keir. I found out that I had received a bit of insurance money from the fire. I hadn't gotten much, but it was enough to pay for boarding school. I wasn't allowed to touch it until my eighteenth birthday, except in the case of education. I was thrilled. Mom encouraged me in this and as soon as my dad found out that I could pay my own way, that it wouldn't be a financial burden to him, he was right behind the idea.

Once accepted into the school, I got all the pertinent information, such as living arrangements and when classes began. I let my family know of my plans. My family at the time included a four-year-old sister, Shauna, and a one-and-a-half-year-old brother, Evan. They probably didn't understand much of what I was saying.

"School starts August 13 and I'll need a ride down with all my things," I told my parents.

Classes didn't actually begin on that date, but all the students were going on an outdoor camping trip as a bonding experience before school began. It was a good way to meet new people.

On August 12, we packed all my things into our big Chevy van and my whole family jumped in, driving the three hours to my new school. Before I knew it, I was standing on campus surveying my new surroundings. Three large buildings were visible from where I stood. Later I found out that that my dorm would be housed in the middle building on the second floor. There were a few classrooms and a small library on the first floor. The third floor housed both the Junior High and Senior High on one end. The younger grades, one through six, were on the other end.

The two buildings on either side of my dorm had multiple functions. One housed the gymnasium and the men's college dorm. The other housed the cafeteria, school office, and women's dorm.

After unloading my suitcases, filled to the brim with clothes and school supplies, my family headed back to the van.

My dad was the last to give me a hug. "We'll be back to pick you up for Christmas," he told me.

And then they were off.

I got a lump in my throat watching the van disappear. Christmas…that seemed like a long ways away. It was not going to be easy being away from home for the first time in my life.

Shortly after my arrival, I was called to the principal's office to fill out some forms. A single page was put before me, with a list of activities on it.

"It's nice to have you at our school, Dave. Your previous grades are quite good and we're excited to see what you can accomplish here. Now, aside from that, you're probably wondering about these papers in front of you. We send students to represent us at Regionals every year in various events. I'd like you to check off the areas you are good at or are interested in."

I looked down at the paper. I saw basketball, volleyball, short plays, singing, essay writing, short story writing…I could shoot a basketball quite well, but I wasn't sure if I could make the team. I didn't circle it. I either had no talent or interest in a lot of the other options.

And then I saw something I was really good at: chess. I circled it.

I slid the list across the table and the principal looked it over.

"Isn't there something else you'd be good at?"

I shook my head.

"How about essay writing? You have quite a life story!" He knew this because I'd had to write a bit about my life to get accepted to the school. "You'd have a good chance of winning just by writing about yourself," he urged.

It didn't really appeal to me, but he convinced me to at least give it a try.

"Okay, good." He checked essay writing on the list, then placed the sheet in my file. "We'll help you to get started on both these events. I'll set you up with a chess instructor and we'll figure out a plan for writing the essay."

They set me up with one of the college students almost immediately and we played a few initial games of chess. I beat him in every one, so the search began for a new chess partner. Once one was located, I played him a few games. He creamed me in every one. He didn't simply beat me; I felt powerless to do anything against him. This wasn't the type of partner I needed, either. I needed someone close to my level but a bit better, to give me the impression that I could win if I applied myself. I found such a player in my third chess partner.

I had excellent teachers and my grades started climbing again. I scored one hundred percent on my very first math exam and the teacher asked if this was common for me. Even though I usually scored in the nineties, I truthfully told her that getting a hundred percent was not a regular occurrence.

I found myself right near the top of the class almost immediately. Over the next couple of years, I competed with two other students, Paul and Elaine, to be the top student.

One term, I won the award for the highest average. It was a good feeling, though I didn't always beat my two closest competitors. I enjoyed getting high marks; it was a way for me to show others that you can't judge a person by their appearance.

Working hard at school kept me somewhat distracted from my mounting homesickness. This was, after all, my first prolonged stay away from home. Before I knew it, Thanksgiving had arrived. Keir was invited to a friend's house for the holiday, along with a few other people, and I was invited as well. It was nice to celebrate Thanksgiving with others.

That first year, I also joined the basketball team, beat most everyone in my school in chess, and used my sense of humor to get a lot of laughs. My humor lay not in telling jokes, but in bouncing funny comments off other people's stories and conversations.

One girl, Lori, took a liking to me and started calling me her hero. I was, at age sixteen, a bit unsure of how to respond to something like that.

She found me in the cafeteria one morning and walked directly over to me.

"How's my hero doing?"

"I'm not sure, I haven't seen him," I replied, trying to be funny. Later I realized that the reply probably hurt her feelings. I was sorry, but it was too late to take it back. I reconnected with her years later and she had no recollection of that event. I apologized anyway.

In the spring, I started coming out of my shell more. Other students noticed before I did, and told me so. I hadn't been aware of it, but they recounted that when I first arrived I looked at the ground wherever I went on campus. Now I was walking around with my head up, looking people in the eye. Obviously I was becoming more confident in myself.

Once I was aware of it, I began paying attention to the changes I saw in myself. I felt free. Change can be a good thing and, in this case, I started loving my new, confident self.

In April, we headed off to Regionals. I was very nervous, not knowing what the competition would be like, especially in an individual event like chess. I had made the basketball team as well and my essay was already written, so I just had to hand it in and wait for the results.

The first morning of Regionals, I played chess and lost. I thought it was all over. The next day, however, I was summoned to play again. I wasn't aware of it, but the rule was that if you lost in the first round to the person who ended up placing first, you got another shot. That's what happened in my case.

The fellow I played next seemed like such a friendly guy that I thought a quick four-move checkmate might catch him off-guard. I tried it, but he blocked me. I then tried a twist, and he went for it. I ended up beating him in six moves.

Because I won that game so quickly, I was immediately set up for another game. If I won this next game, I'd come in second place; if I lost, I'd be third. It was getting late and I'd been up since the crack of dawn. The sharpness of my game was starting to dwindle the later it got.

We were down to our last few men and my opponent had the upper hand. When I was down to just my king, he was down to a king and a rook, as I remember it. Well, I went for a stalemate, which would mean a draw: no one would win and we'd have to play again the following day.

The rule in chess is that once your opponent has you down to just your king, he has twenty-five moves in which to checkmate you. Twenty-five moves for each opponent: fifty moves in total. Well, I purposely moved my king in a way that did not cooperate with where he needed me to move. I'm sure my opponent was getting tired as well, because the game ended in a draw.

The next morning, refreshed from a night of sleep, I won quite easily, placing me second overall. The experience was nerve-wracking and my arm had developed a tick. A vein jumped in my forearm and I spent a couple of games watching the sleeve of my shirt moving up and down to the rhythm of my heartbeat…

Our basketball team also placed in the top three, and I won first place in essay writing!

CHAPTER 18

YOU'RE MY HERO!

Dave, Ages 16–18

I had a tough time being away from home that first year of boarding school. The homesickness made me feel the effects of my appearance even more. By midyear, a lot of students were dating. Not everyone, but most. My friends were also dating, so I didn't get to hang out with them as much as I wanted. It could be quite lonely. Granted, I was shy. As a young man, I wanted a girl by my side just the same as any other guy my age. Put together, these things put me under a great emotional strain.

I was friends with many girls, but they weren't interested in me romantically. On the weekends, when the couples disappeared and friends planned trips into the city, I often found myself alone. I started getting depressed a lot. So much so that I developed an ulcer. With the added stress of chess, it was almost too much for me.

Compared to the other students, I was sick in bed a lot. Yet through all this, I managed to maintain high grades. Academics were important to me, because they countered my perception that others viewed me as mentally slow because of my appearance. My grades represented concrete proof that I wasn't.

I got depressed when I was alone, but the rest of the time I was my happy, funny self. In talking years later with some of the students, they recalled that I was the life of the party. They remembered that everyone cheered up when I entered the room and laughed all the time because I was so funny.

I would sometimes have to stand up in class to read a report I'd written; the students doubled over, holding their sides in laughter. This started irritating me so much that one day, when a few of my peers where laughing at my speech on bears or some other topic, I stopped and asked, "What's so funny?" My report was serious and I couldn't understand why they were laughing.

One of them answered, "It's not the report that's funny; it's how you say it."

It still wasn't clear to me why they were laughing so hard, but whatever! It seems my sense of humor came out even when I was being serious!

Like all things, the year finally came to an end. I was more confident and comfortable with myself at the end than I'd been at the beginning. So off I headed for home and a summer of relaxing and hanging out with friends.

Near the end of the summer, I went to get my learner's license. I was a little older than most teens because my dad wouldn't let me practice in any of the family vehicles. I passed the exam and received my learner's license without any problems. My full driver's license would have to wait until the following summer. Being away at school, I wouldn't have the means or the time to do it any sooner.

When I returned to school for Grade Eleven, we again began practicing for Regionals where I'd be participating in the same events: chess, essay writing, and basketball. When Regionals started, I played chess the first morning and won, followed by a couple more wins.

Then I met my fourth opponent. My mentors had cautioned me never to take my queen out too early in the game, but I had and now she was in trouble. I sat wracking my brain, trying to find a way out of my predicament. I didn't want to lose my queen, because if I lost her I would be hard-pressed to win against a good opponent.

Some spectators were walking around watching us play. Suddenly, a girl from my school named Sandy was standing by our table. I looked up at her inquisitively, my brain still deep in the game.

"You'll win," she said.

"Really? How do you know?"

"Because you're my hero!"

That touched my heart. I couldn't very well let her down, could I? But she probably had no idea what sort of bind I was in. I searched the chessboard with renewed vigor and suddenly saw something I hadn't seen before. I saw a way to win. To do it, though, I had to play one of my other men as a decoy. The piece my opponent would have to use to take out my decoy would open the door for me to checkmate him with my queen. My heart was thudding in my chest as I tried, as casually as I could, to move my chess piece.

Would he see the trap or would he go for it? He went for it and took my unprotected decoy! I quickly pounced and put him in checkmate. I'd won!

My final game was the gold medal round. My opponent looked like a genius. I was scared to death. We fought long and hard before, even though I had fewer men than him, I saw it—a way to beat him. It would only take three moves as long as he moved where I figured he would. It worked, and I won!

At the end, though, he wanted to take back those last three moves and see if he could beat me. We called the referee over to let him know who had won and what we were doing. As soon as I had won, all the strain and tension left my body and we took back those last three moves and started again. I crushed him. This opened my eyes to how well I could play if I didn't let my nerves affect my game.

I had won my first gold medal playing chess, but it was the final year I played because the strain to my body was too much. I couldn't eat or sleep well and the ticks continued to spring up on my arm. I made the wise choice to retire from competitive chess.

At the end of the three days of Regionals, all the awards were handed out in front of the student body. As I went up front to collect my gold medal for chess, all of the students rose to their feet, giving me a standing ovation. There was nothing quite like having so many people be so supportive of my win. It was overwhelming and I felt taller the further down the aisle I got. It almost made me feel invincible, stronger than I really was.

I received a medal for basketball, too, in addition to being named the first place winner of essay writing. Again the students stood to their feet, clapping thunderously as I walked to the stage to receive my medal.

Years later, I found out that Elaine, one of the students, remembered me as being fiercely competitive, not just for the highest marks but in everything I did. She remembered a time when I climbed the peg board in the gym. It was attached to the side of the wall and the bottom of the board was about six feet off the ground. There were two pegs, and the goal was to climb the board by placing the pegs into the holes, using them as leverage to pull yourself up. It took a lot of strength. After reaching the top, you would come back down the same way you went up. Elaine remembered that the only reason I mastered the peg board was because it was in the school and I had been determined not to leave anything in the school undone.

I didn't see myself as competitive all the time, but I knew I could be that way. This was most evident on a forty-kilometer walk (just short of a marathon) I went on with others from my school. I was walking with Cheri, a friend, for the first few miles before I noticed that the group of people who had taken off running earlier were now out of sight on the road. I couldn't stop thinking how far ahead they were getting.

I walked with Cheri until I couldn't take it anymore. I told her I was going to take off and catch up to the front-runners, which I did. I think I came in third. I was so dead tired that night and my legs were so weak that I had a hard time climbing onto my top bunk. I had completed the distance in just over seven hours, not bad considering I'd started with no intention of racing.

In the awards department, there was one particular award I won every year: fewest demerits. Demerits were given when school rules were broken, and unlike my private school back home, I never broke any. I won this award almost every semester, and therefore won all three years of high school.

No one called me a Goody Two-Shoes, though. Maybe it was because I was well-liked and funny, or maybe it was because students saw that award as a good one to win. Granted, I did attend a small school of only one hundred students or so, but it was still hard to place on top in any area. For the least demerits award, for example, I had a total of seven demerits over the three years of high school. This was the same amount some students got in a day.

Some would say I won some awards because I was well-liked by staff and got away with things. There may be some truth to that.

One fellow, Russ, sat beside me in class and tried to help me get some demerits. You could get a demerit for talking in class or passing notes. Russ was constantly passing me notes and whispering to me while I did my best to ignore him. Eventually the teacher would appear beside us, just as Russ had done one of these things.

Great, I'd think. *I hadn't done anything and now I'm going to get demerits.* But the teacher seemed to always know what was happening and Russ got the demerits. Once he had amassed a pile of demerits, he grew tired of his game.

Demerits were not just given out in school, but also on campus for breaking campus rules. One of these rules was no water fights. Some exceptions were made on hot days, but water fights were never allowed inside the buildings, where they caused the most damage.

I was involved in a water fight once in the school kitchen. As a campus resident, I and eight other students had kitchen duties after each meal. I cleaned pots and pans with another fellow. He washed and I rinsed, dried, and put them away. When the water fight broke out, I went for the best weapon: the spray hose used to spray the plates down before washing them, and I promptly hosed everyone down.

The water fight didn't last long, since everyone was drenched in a matter of minutes. I had just turned away from the entrance to the kitchen and was leaning over the pots and pans area when the school president walked in. He was livid and gave us all a lecture. During the whole episode, I kept working and drying the pots. Everyone except me was standing near the kitchen entrance when we got caught. We were all dripping wet, but I had my back to the president. It suddenly occurred to me that although the front of me was soaked, the back of me—the only part he could see—was completely dry.

We all expected to get demerits, mostly because the school president said we'd get them. I ended up not getting any and I can only surmise it was because it looked like I was innocently working.

One time, I came back from town on a Friday night and was late for curfew. If I was caught, I'd get five demerits. Every ten earned in a school year resulted in having to work on a Saturday: a student's sacred day off. I knew of a footpath that skirted the front gate, which was locked. I had taken this path in my car a couple of times, so I knew I could get through. The gate was originally installed to deter boys from the local town from driving onto campus late at night.

I slowly eased my car onto the path, bumping over rocks and roots, my side mirrors scraping the trees on either side of my car. Eventually I made it through, having to pass a few staff residences to get to my dorm. As I drove by the first place, I saw the caretaker's wife peering out the front window. My heart almost stopped. Surely she recognized my car!

She didn't come out of her house and I made it back to the dorm and into my bed with no further scares. For the next three days, I fully expected to find those demerits in my mailbox or for one of the faculty to pull me aside, but I never heard a thing about it. I also didn't try that path again in my car. I didn't think my heart could take it!

To the natural eye, it didn't look like there was much to me either mentally or physically. I had a slim, wiry build, yet I liked to wrestle, to show that I wasn't a weakling. One of my favorite things to do was wrestle around with the guys who weighed over two hundred pounds. There were only two students I did this with: one was two hundred pounds even, named Paul, and the other was two hundred and ten pounds. I'd wrap my arms around their waists and lift them off the ground. I weighed in at one hundred and ten.

One day I was wrestling the two-tenner. We were out in the schoolyard and ended up on the grass on our backs.

I reached over, grabbed a hold of him, and made the mistake of rolling him over top of me. I heard a few popping sounds that couldn't have been good. As long as we stayed on our feet, I was fine picking these guys up. I never tried this other move again.

I was over at Paul's house once and we horsed around in his older brother's room. I was lying across the bed when Paul leaped in the air right at me! I raised my knee to protect my chest, and when he landed on it I swung my leg up, using his momentum to help me. He flew right over me and landed on the floor on the other side of the bed. Luckily he wasn't hurt and we all got a good laugh at how ridiculous he'd looked flying over my head.

In the summertime, I headed back home. Among other things, I planned to get my full driver's license. My mom and dad insisted that I take driver training, and we were thrilled when my mom discovered I could get it for free at the Glenrose, since I was handicapped. My friends were livid when they found out I got my training for free.

CHAPTER 19

....

CAMP

Dave, Ages 19–20

I had not yet learned the full extent of what I was capable of with my hands, so it was good that I went to the Glenrose for my driver's training. That way, if I needed anything to help me drive, they could provide it.

I was confident that I would not need any adaptors in the car to help me grasp the steering wheel. I didn't want any special attachments, because then I'd always be limited to driving my own car. As it turned out, I didn't need anything special. In fact, there was a knob attached to the steering wheel for another student and it was constantly getting in my way.

While taking the in-car sessions, my confidence grew; when my dad saw this, he took me car shopping. I did things a bit backwards: I bought a car before I had my license. I finished the course, then set up an appointment to take my driving test.

I used the Glenrose's driver training car to take my test. This car was big and long, but I was used to it. My driver's education instructor drove me over to the motor vehicle office to take my road test. She waited inside the building while I took off on my road exam. The exam went smoothly, but when it was over there were a few tense moments. I had to sit and wait while the examiner wrote on her clipboard. I was nervous, but then she finally turned to me and told me how I'd done.

"You did well but were a bit hesitant at times. You have a good grip on the steering wheel, so I don't think you'll need any attachments put on to help you drive." She gave me a big smile. "Congratulations, Dave. You pass! The only thing is that I don't think you'll be able to handle a standard transmission, so I'm going to put that restriction on your license."

I was a bit stunned. How could she tell I wouldn't be able to drive a stick shift? I didn't want to argue, in case she told me the only way to get a license without the restriction was to come back and retake the test with a standard transmission vehicle. I didn't want her to put my license on hold. I wanted it today! There was no way I had the time to learn how to drive a stick shift before school started again, and there wasn't a stick shift at my driver education school at the Glenrose. My parents had one, but they wanted me to have some training and experience before they let me drive it. I kept my mouth shut and accepted the license.

I resented the restriction on my license. I didn't like anyone telling me what I was or wasn't capable of doing. I did find out that to have the restriction taken off, coming back in a standard transmission vehicle and retaking the test would be necessary. I kept that in the back of my mind for the future, since I'd already purchased a car with an automatic transmission.

I didn't take the car back to school with me in the fall, but I did take it after Christmas. I didn't feel ready to drive in the snow and ice, so I waited until spring to drive.

After a couple months behind the wheel, I was driving like a manic. I liked to go fast and I had miles and miles of country highway to practice on.

Grad was right around the corner, and I was looking forward to finally being finished high school. As exciting as my three years at boarding school had been, I couldn't wait to be finished. Summer couldn't come fast enough for me.

School tradition was to have a big graduation night, where the grads were all seated in the decorated cafeteria and served by other students. I asked Elaine to be my date, and she accepted.

The day before grad, I was in the school office helping another student with a job we'd been given. Suddenly I became aware of someone hollering outside. I peered out of the third-floor window and looked down. There, at a full sprint, was my now seven-year-old sister Shauna screaming my name at the top of her lungs.

"Who is that?" my classmate demanded.

"My sister. I'd better go down and get her before she disturbs the whole campus. She gets a little excited at the thought of seeing me."

My whole family had come to watch me cross the stage and accept my high school diploma, except for Keir, who had moved to Ontario and was unable to come out.

The next day was graduation day, and I was excited! All the grads had seats on the stage. There weren't that many of us, so we all fit. My dad took pictures that day, and in one you can see me sitting on the stage with the rest of the grads looking innocent. Seated beside me was Elaine, her face turned towards me, laughing at something I'd just said.

My fellow classmates remember me as being quite out-going, and yet those were lonely years. However, I would never trade them away. Those were the years when I started to grow out of my shyness and learn who I was.

*   *   *

After high school, I went to the college on the same campus. The money I'd received from the fire paid my way. My plan was to go for one year and then see where I wanted to go from there.

For my first year of college, I lived on campus with the school staff. That wasn't my first time living with staff, as I had done it during my senior year of high school as well. The difference was that in high school I had lived with the *college* staff. Now that I was in college, I lived with the *high school* staff. I didn't want to live with one of my own teachers, because I didn't want them to know my study habits.

I didn't study all the time and I liked to start late in the evening. If I lived with one of my teachers, they would always know when I had an exam. So if I was relaxing in their living room, I didn't want them asking me when I was going to start studying. I didn't need any extra pressure!

In college, I continued to get good grades, which I hadn't expected. I'd gotten top grades in high school, but I still didn't believe that I was smart enough to excel just anywhere. I was nervous about going to college. My parents encouraged me to relax and told me I'd be fine.

They were right; I continued to do well and was near the top of the class. I tended to do better on the exams that I had heard were very hard; they scared me, so I studied like a maniac and usually got very high grades. On the other hand, I tended to get lower grades on the exams I had heard were easy.

I liked to joke around about my marks. Often, after a really tough exam, I'd talk with the other students about how they thought they'd done. They'd answer, and then ask, "How did you do?"

I'd put on a straight face and say in a sad voice, "I think…I think I failed…"

When we got back our marks, some of the girls would be concerned and gather around me. "How did you do?" one of them would ask.

"I did okay. Better than I thought, anyway."

"But what did you get?"

I didn't always want to tell them, especially if I had done really well. With the right gal, though, I'd tell her and then she'd smoke me in the arm—usually because I'd gotten a ninety-five or ninety-eight. I never let those high grades go to my head, however, and I didn't like rubbing it in. But I did like to joke around with it.

I was a good student, good at sports and track, and I was a decent chess player. As good as I was at these things, I tried hard not to let it go to my head. I didn't like to brag about my accomplishments. It was easy to brag, but harder not to. I tried to take the harder road.

I loved to see people smile and hear them laugh. One of my favorite things to do was to fill in the blank when others couldn't finish a sentence. I'd fill in the blank with a silly word or phrase to get a laugh. I also relied on my humor to get me through the tough times.

One of my friends once tried to tell me about a really nice gift her husband's company had givne him when he resigned. She said, "It was a really nice…really nice portrait of…of…" She couldn't think of the right word.

"His boss's dog?" I suggested.

She laughed.

In March of my freshman year, I found out about an annual school tradition where the college population was broken up into teams and sent out to different provinces and states in Canada and the United States. The idea was that each team would go out to different venues and sing, perform short skits or plays that we'd learned, and then take turns talking about our lives: what we'd gone through, where we'd come from, etc. I ended up on the same team as my friend Tim.

We were at a new place almost every night, so each night one person shared his or her life story. We constantly rotated. As soon as I shared about my life, the whole team voted that my story had the most impact and should be shared every night.

I didn't enjoy speaking and felt that the rest of the team didn't, either, and were using me as an excuse not to do it. I wasn't too impressed, but I did it anyway. I actually grew more comfortable speaking, and by the end of the tour saw it as a great opportunity and honor. I had a great time on the three-week tour. When we came back, we had just over a month until the end of the college term.

That summer, I drove forty-five hours with Tim, Keir, and a few other friends to attend a friend's wedding in Ontario. Keir had flown to Alberta to visit the family and now he was catching a ride back. There were six of us travelling in two cars. By switching drivers, we drove straight through, only stopping for gas and food.

The groom had been my roommate during my second year of high school. We'd had a common love of chess and played together constantly. We even set up an ongoing game of chess in our room. We checked the board each time we came in. If a move had been made, we would take our turn. Playing chess this way often took us days. We would play game after game like this, because we were on different schedules and neither of us had the spare hours to sit down for a drawn-out game.

Before I headed east that summer, I counseled at a camp in Saskatchewan for a month. I grew quite attached to some of the kids there. For the most part, all the kids in my cabin were good-natured and well-behaved. I was the kind of counselor the kids couldn't take advantage of or run rampant on. I was firm and tough when I needed to be, yet we had a lot of fun.

I had a new group of kids every week. One week, I counseled a young guy named Lyle, who was about twelve, smaller, and more timid than the other boys. They tried to take advantage of him, pestering him to see how far they could push him. Until I stepped in, that is. I didn't appreciate people ganging up on one person, and I was willing to tackle the whole lot of them. After speaking my piece, they knew where I stood!

I told them that if they really wanted to pick on someone, they could try picking on me. They didn't take me up on the offer, but they did ease off on Lyle. I didn't expect them to totally back off, otherwise how would Lyle learn to stand up for himself? The way Lyle reacted to having me stand up for him led me to believe that he didn't often have someone to intercede on his behalf. He seemed to appreciate it. I really liked him and wanted to give him a little breathing room to just enjoy camp.

During the first week of camp, I counseled eleven- and twelve year-olds, but by my last week I was counseling fifteen- to eighteen year-olds. I was only twenty myself, so when I had the older boys in my cabin I never told them my age; I thought it might cause problems for them to know I was only a couple years older than them.

I counseled a boy with Down Syndrome during my last week. I got the impression that he felt he could get away with a lot because of his condition. I was convinced others let him get away with things because they thought he didn't know any better. I had no intention of letting him get away with this.

I knew he could understand me. When I told him not to do something, he would ignore me, but when I informed him of his punishment, he got mad. I had told him a few times to stop borrowing the other boys' things or eating the snacks they kept by their bed. He ignored everything I said, so I finally told him he would get no snacks from the canteen that night.

We were in the cabin when I laid down the rules. He looked me over as if sizing me up, then suddenly took off running for the canteen. This act reinforced my belief that he understood more than he was letting on. I ran after him and easily kept pace. I didn't feel the need to get to the canteen before him, because when he got there he got into line while I went right to the counter and told the counselors he wasn't allowed to buy snacks that evening.

After that, I backed off and just watched. He looked triumphant when he got up to the counter, but that quickly faded when he found out I'd already put a stop to him. After that episode, we seemed to reach an understanding.

I had begun to learn at the Glenrose that outward appearances can be deceiving. Many students didn't look like they had much promise, but that wasn't always the case. It was hard to tell just by looking at them, but a few had very sharp minds. Some students had muscular diseases which could affect their speech, so they were sometimes hesitant to try communicating. Others had a slack, blank face and looked like their minds were empty. I learned I had to wait and see what they were really like.

These lessons taught me not to make assumptions. By waiting, I could better gauge what a person was like. My appearance certainly didn't show what I was capable of, and the same was true of others I ran into people when I was young who thought I had learning disabilities because of my burns. They would talk to me slowly, as if I didn't understand English.

CHAPTER 20

....

DRAMA TEAM

Dave, Ages 20–21

When the summer ended, I went back for a second year of college. Unlike the past two years, I moved back into the student dorm. I was welcome to continue living with the staff, but I thought this might be my last year there and wanted to experience dorm life again.

I was never excited about school. Although I always seemed to do well academically, I was never one to look forward to school and was always glad when another year came to a close. At the same time, when the year was over and all the students (who had become like family to me) left, I felt like a part of me left with them.

On weekends, I often went into town with a friend or two. I noticed that even when I was well into my twenties, people still stared at me. Usually it was just looks, but sometimes it was more. For example, if I walked up to a counter without the cashier seeing me, they would sometimes gasp when I appeared in front of them. If they saw me coming, the few seconds they had to prepare themselves seemed to help. As I grew a bit older, it either stopped happening or I no longer noticed it.

The last time I was asked why I was wearing a mask was in the winter when my car got stuck in the snow. The road had just enough of a slope that it was impossible to get out. A fellow stopped by to help, but he couldn't push me out by himself, even with both of us rocking the car back and forth. We needed one more person. Soon, a second man showed up. He lived across the street. As he walked over, he asked, "You need a hand pushing?" He caught his first glimpse of me as I got out of my car and stood up.

"Why are you wearing a mask?" he inquired, sounding more curious than anything.

This put me at ease. I was tired, it was past midnight, and it had been a long week. All I had in me was to tell the basic truth. "I'm not. I was burned in a fire."

"I'm sorry, man. I couldn't see too well in this light."

It amazed me why some people stared and got scared when they saw me while others came right up and talked to me, their eyes open and friendly as if I was no different than anyone else. What was it about this latter group of strangers that allowed them to see beyond the scars and see me as just another person?

Throughout my life, I've come to see pity in the eyes of many. I never saw it in my family, though. They always saw more ability and talent in me than I saw in myself, and pushed me towards it. In time, I began to see myself through their eyes and this attitude change allowed my talents to flourish.

*   *   *

My second year of college was a little tougher, so I had to study hard. I preferred to begin my studying around one or two o'clock in the morning, go for a couple hours, then sleep and get up at 7:30 for breakfast. By the week's end, I was exhausted. I would sleep in on Saturday, often skipping breakfast. I loved my food, so this was a big sacrifice for me.

When class ended for lunch, I was often the first out the door, through the building, and down the sidewalk to the cafeteria. Even if I wasn't the first one out the door, I passed whoever was in front of me, sprinting as fast as I could to get to the front of the cafeteria line.

One evening, on a rare day when I had started studying early, I heard a major water fight going on out in the hall. I took a peek out of my room and saw that the Resident Assistant (RA) was right in the thick of things. The RA had been picked by the college staff to ensure things didn't get out of hand.

I had no interest in getting wet that night, so I went back to my studying. After all, I had an exam the next day.

About an hour or so later, someone knocked on my door. When I opened it, I found out that the water fight had created large puddles on the carpet and the fellow at my door wanted my help to figure out what to do.

They had to get things cleaned up before the evening staff completed their nightly walkthrough and locked the dorm up for the night. The carpet was so soggy that it made wet sucking sounds when you stepped on it.

I told them to get towels, place them on the wet areas, and stand on them to soak up the water faster. They did this until someone could walk over the spot without it making a sound. Next, I instructed them to unscrew the light bulbs above the wet spots, thus rendering the dark spot on the carpet invisible.

The test came when the fellow who was on lockup duty came into our dorm, said goodnight to those he saw, and walked the entire length of the hall, disappearing out the back door. Everyone was holding their breath.

He hadn't noticed a thing. I don't know why the student came to me for help, but it made me feel needed. It was a nice feeling.

Certain periods of my life shaped me in different ways. I had plenty of solitude, time spent in thought or reflection apart from my peers. I often read when I was alone, and when I was younger I created new things with Lego. I didn't build set objects; I created objects out of my imagination. The solitude made me a thinker. The periods I spent in the hospital hardened my resolve and made me a fighter.

These attributes had always been part of me, but the incredible pain in my young life brought them out sooner and raised them to heights I never would have experienced otherwise.

Even though my resolve was deep, there were still some things that felt like too much for me. At one point in college, I felt overwhelmed by all the work expected of me. Since I had a track record for academic excellence, the college administration talked me out of taking easy electives and I took their advice.

After a while, my responsibilities piled up and it seemed too much for me to bear at age twenty. It felt like a crushing weight on my back. For some reason, a verse from the Bible started running through my mind: *"Call to Me, and I will answer you, and show you great and mighty things, which you do not know"* (Jeremiah 33:3). That night, I called out to God and the huge weight lifted and was gone. Just like that. That was the moment God became real to me. Before that moment, I had thought of him as being millions of miles away.

After that year's Christmas break, our RA informed us that he was leaving and two new RAs would be selected. My dorm mate Dave and I were selected.

It was amazing how many Daves attended my college, particularly since the population of our college and high school totaled less than two hundred people any given year. At one point, there were six Daves. That was such a large number compared to other years. One time during a meal in the cafeteria, someone asked all the Daves to stand. We promptly stood, along with a few other students just trying to be funny.

In college, I continued to let my own brand of humor run full force. I sat beside a few girls who loved my sense of humor, and I would pass notes to them during class. Sometimes they would burst out laughing when they read my words, drawing unwanted attention to themselves. At these times, I would sit unmoving in my chair, looking innocent. The girls always let me know after class it was my fault, but they were never mad.

Though I was the funny guy in college, I shut my sense of humor down later in life because I found I was not being taken seriously. I did have a serious side, but not many saw it because my humor naturally came out first. It has taken years for me to learn a balance between my humorous and serious sides.

After graduation, I found out that a few students were planning to set up a drama team the following year. Their plan was to tour around Canada, the U.S., and part of Mexico. As soon as I heard about it, I knew it was for me and I let it be known that I was interested.

I spent the summer after graduation working for a family that sold their own vegetables at a market garden. I weeded by hoe and tractor for a few weeks. One day while weeding, I re-pulled a muscle I had hurt playing soccer years before. The chiropractor at the time had told me the affected muscle was a tiny one in my lower back.

This pulled muscle rendered me nearly useless. It hurt to walk or move my arms. It hurt sitting, standing, or lying down. I could not find any peace from the pain. I tried working through the intense pain and spent my breaks lying flat out on the grass, trying to recover. My boss noticed this after two days and we agreed it was best that I throw in the towel. My back wasn't going to heal if I continued to work. I stayed with a family nearby and was in no hurry to head back home, so I hung around visiting friends.

One night, at 1:30 a.m., I was driving back to my place down a country highway on a dark, moonless night. Coming up over a hill, I saw something big lying on the highway immediately in front of my car. There was no way to avoid it, and just as I recognized what it was...SMASH! It all happened in a split second. I had no time to react.

I hit the dark shape and my car flipped over onto its roof, careening down the highway. My car hurtled through the night, leaving behind it a trail of sparks. I couldn't see anything and had no idea what I was heading towards. It was terrifying. I called out to God for help. My mind finally registered what I had hit—a black cow. According to the police, I had knocked the cow eighty yards down the road and my car slid a hundred yards on its roof. Talk about a touchdown!

After the car came to a stop, I unbuckled my seatbelt, fell down to the roof of my upside-down car, and crawled out through the side window, which had been smashed out.

I stood for a moment as my heart started to slow down from its jackhammer pace. My mind was calm now that my car had come to a stop, and I had one thought: to walk back to my friend's house. I'd only left there ten minutes earlier so I was sure they wouldn't be asleep yet.

It was so dark as I walked back up the highway that I couldn't tell where the road ended and the ditch began. I soon came to a spot on the highway that was darker than the night. It was the black cow.

It wasn't until the next day that I saw the devastation of that crash. The contents of my car, the windshield, and various other car parts were strewn up and down the ditch. I knew then how fortunate I'd been when I saw three power poles by the side of the road that my car had slid harmlessly past.

I only walked a few minutes down the road before a car stopped and the driver offered to take me to my friend's house a few miles up the road. When I walked in the door, my friends took one look at the blood running down my forehead and drove me to the nearest hospital about twenty minutes away.

CHAPTER 21

....

DRIVING A STICK SHIFT

Dave, Ages 21–25

I was fine as far as the hospital staff could tell. In fact, they commented that I was more alert than they were as I corrected a couple discrepancies on their forms. The wounds were shallow cuts and abrasions, probably from flying glass when my side window had exploded. They cleaned the wounds, bandaged them up, and sent me off. Other than a few cuts and scrapes, the only side effect was neck pain which lasted a couple of months, and of course my car was completely totaled.

My dad drove five hours to get me and take me home. In the fall, I was back in full health, so I headed off to join the drama team.

Once I was back on campus, we started practicing right away. The first order of business was picking the plays we would perform and then assigning parts. I enjoyed the humorous plays the most, because I loved making people laugh.

We often practiced in front of the staff and students before hitting the road. Even though we'd perform a short play they'd seen numerous times, my parts rarely failed to get a laugh out of them.

Only six people signed up for the drama team and everyone was a good fit, so we were set. We called ourselves the SALT team. Some of the students nicknamed us the Assault Team. We started practicing in September, the same time classes started, and after a month we headed out on the road. We toured Alberta and Saskatchewan until Christmas. Then, after a two-week break, we headed straight to Corpus Christie, Texas, where we stayed with the families of some of the team members.

From there, we hopped down into Mexico, where we spent two weeks at a local mission doing mime (because of the language barrier). After the show, I would share my story through a translator.

When our time there came to an end, we packed our touring van and headed back to Texas. We headed north and only had a few stops before entering back into Canada through Ontario. I shared my life story over a hundred times that year.

We arrived back at college about a month before the end of the term and helped set up that year's semi-annual youth retreat, where teens from all over Western Canada came to experience a bit of campus life for three days. They would eat cafeteria food, sleep in dorm rooms, and be entertained by the students on stage. Our drama team also performed a few plays.

All in all, it was quite a year. We put about nine thousand miles on a beat up Dodge Ram van and experienced many unforgettable moments. Some of the strong bonds we forged would last a lifetime.

When the year was over, we all went our separate ways. It was heart-wrenching for me to know I wouldn't be seeing these friends every day from then on. Many had become as close as family.

I stayed on campus a bit longer and ended up buying another car, one with manual transmission. I didn't appreciate having the restriction on my license, so I set out to have it removed by learning to drive a stick shift.

Although I wasn't allowed to drive such a car, it was okay while I was on private property—in other words, on campus. It only took a few weeks to feel comfortable with the clutch, gear shift, and coordination of the clutch with the gas pedal. From time to time, I would stall when coming to a complete stop, but I soon mastered that, too. Then I headed home to complete my mission. I brought a friend of mine to drive me and the car home, after which I immediately began to see about getting the restriction lifted.

I booked another road test. At the end of the session I thought I drove well, but the instructor told me that though

I could handle a stick shift fine, I was a bit aggressive on my lane changes and turns.

"But that's not what we're here to test," she said. "Congratulations! I'll have this restriction taken off for you." We headed into the motor vehicle office and within a few minutes I had a restriction-free license! I'd achieved victory.

I was home, finished college, and had a year of travelling under my belt. Now it was time for me to sit down and determine where I was going next in life. I decided to head to university and finish my degree. In talking with a few friends who also wanted to go to university, we decided to go to the same one. Now it was just a matter of figuring out *which* one.

After much discussion, we settled on Edmonton, Alberta. This was nice for me, since my family would be close, even though I did not intend to live at home. Four of us came to Edmonton to attend university and two other friends wound up there for work. In total, there were three guys and three girls in our group. We decided to get neighboring apartments close to the university, one for the guys and one for the girls.

At university, I again had my usual concerns about academics, but I also had a new concern: I assumed the exams would be longer here and wondered if I'd be able to write fast enough to finish in the allotted time.

I needn't have worried, because I did fine in the first semester and felt confidant heading into the second. My friends and I, having already experienced campus life, all lived off-campus and wanted to experience the freedom of the city.

I didn't look for a job that first year because I wanted to see how I fared academically. Since I did very well, immediately after spring finals I began looking for a part-time job. In the first month, I sent out ninety résumés and had dozens of interviews, but my appearance was a huge hurdle to overcome. When I walked through the door, the interview would often begin and end this way: "I don't think you can do this job."

I began to think I'd never get hired.

In the midst of my search, a friend of mine called me up and said he was working in a call center and his company was hiring. It was a sales position and it didn't sound too bad. They didn't do cold calling (calling from the phone book), so I applied.

"What sort of sales experience do you have?" I was asked in the interview.

I didn't have any, but I put up a brave front and told them that my sales experience was selling myself everywhere I went. This was true, since I had been trying to convince people my whole life that I could do anything.

I found out later that my friend was called into the office after my interview.

"Can he even dial a phone?"

"Of course he can!" he told his bosses.

I was called back for a second interview, completed it, then went home and waited. I didn't hear anything after a couple of days, so I went back to sending out résumés.

The next day, I got the call. I was hired!

Within a month, I was doing so well that my boss came to talk to me.

"We hope you stay here until you retire!"

Since I'd had such great feedback, I thought I'd ask for a big favor: a week off in August. My whole family was going camping that week and I really wanted to join them.

"We don't normally do this," my boss said, "but for you…okay!"

The company didn't grant any vacation time until they had worked for a full year, so they really were making an exception for me. I couldn't quite believe it, but I was glad to have a week off with my family in the mountains.

I continued working at the call center when I returned to school in the fall, working twenty hours a week on top of a full course load.

After university graduation, I had one final major surgery: a skin graft on my head. Skin was taken off my right leg from an area about four or five inches long just below the knee, and applied to my scalp. After the surgery, the doctor told me that baseball caps were too abrasive on my scalp, so I had to find something else to wear. I thought of a bandana, which I'd seen some men wear. To this day, I've never worn a baseball cap again.

*   *   *

All the things I had to go through sometimes made me feel sorry for myself. It was in high school when I first started feeling self-pity. I hated the feeling. Self-pity came down so many paths. I wanted for others to come and help me, to be around me when I needed them. But letting myself go down those paths only made me feel mad. I felt even sorrier for myself when they didn't happen the way I wanted them to.

Self-pity would manifest itself in everyday ways. For example, I'd get mad at my roommate for not being there to give my car a boost when it wouldn't start. Without self-pity, I would have just called someone to help me.

Along those same lines, I'd wish people were always around to help with anything I required. But this, of course, never actually helped me get things done. I'd need a ride somewhere, need help putting something together at home, or simply want help with a random problem. Instead of wishing, I should have just tackled the problem at hand.

Self-pity also reared its ugly head when I threw pity parties. My friends would come over and try to cheer me up, inviting me to do something with them, but I would continually turn them away.

Once they left, I would be angry at them for not trying harder…and also angry at myself for not going. That was a major lose-lose situation, because I'd fall even deeper into my pity party and have fewer resources to get out of it. Self-pity was so debilitating in my earlier years that it rendered me helpless. Though I would desperately want to go out and do something with friends, I often couldn't bring myself to.

Sometimes in stores, when my wallet was on the counter, I would suddenly find myself wondering what I would do if someone grabbed it and ran. I'd look around the vicinity and size people up to see who might help me chase the thief down. Self-pity was the same for me as feeling sick and just wanting someone to take care of me. Except for one big difference: self-pity was a choice and being sick was not.

I thought I had gotten rid of self-pity in high school. Then, years later, I found myself with tears running down my face for no reason one night. I thought I was losing it. When it suddenly occurred to me that it was self-pity, it was quite a blow. I could now see that I hadn't gotten rid of it…I just hadn't recognized it.

It took me years to recognize all the disguises of self-pity. Many times I just felt like crying over all I've had to go through. This made it tough to get anything done, wishing others would help me or convince me they really wanted to hang out with me.

I once told an acquaintance that I loved going camping but didn't get to go as much as I would have liked because I didn't know many people who liked to camp.

"Next time my wife and I go, you'll have to come with us," he kindly told me.

Yeah right, I thought with a twinge in my heart. That was self-pity, trying to limit me once again.

At times, I was so focused on wanting a girlfriend that I couldn't receive the love of those around me—because it wasn't the type of love I was looking for.

I finally got rid of self-pity by confronting my attitude that I wasn't worth loving. I had to deal with my feelings of loneliness. Self-pity would still come, and I'd get stuck again if I entertained the thoughts. Instead, I refused to entertain thoughts of self-pity anymore.

CHAPTER 22

···

PUBLIC SPEAKING

Dave

My life was changed forever, all because of a practical joke. Jokes can seem so harmless, but my story reveals just how wrong they can go.

It wasn't until a few years after the fire that I learned what happened to Beth, Kay, and Scott and Bernice. They went to the local hospital the same night that Keir and I did. Kat had first, second, and third-degree burns on her back, neck, both hands, and throat, under her left arm, and the front of her left leg from the knee to her hip. The burns needed to be treated, but she did not require surgery. Kat was in the hospital one month before being released.

Kat had initially invited just Beth to her backyard sleepover. Then, when our family moved in next door, she invited my sister Kimberly, too. Beth and Kimberly died that night and Keir and I both wound up in the hospital in critical condition. The feeling of responsibility Kat had for all this pain must have been overwhelming. I personally never felt she was in any way to blame for that night.

Kat's father, Scott, spent two weeks in the hospital. His feet had both been badly burned from jumping into the fire to save everyone. Two weeks after his release from the hospital, he returned to work. Scott had burns on both hands and his right hand was particularly bad. He had burns going up his right leg past his knee, and also burn spots on his hip and right forearm.

Four months after the fire, Scott didn't think any of his injuries would interfere with his work, but his feet were never quite normal again and were always uncomfortable in hot weather.

Kat's mom suffered second-degree burns on her hands, causing them to blister. She received her burns from trying to put out the fire on Kat's and Keir's pajamas.

I heard that one of the boys who had thrown firecrackers in the tent suffered years of remorse. Kat told me that for years she couldn't go by the old neighborhood without feeling like retching. She could still hear everyone she had invited screaming that night. The sounds and smells from that night stayed with her.

What happened to me in the fire dominated my life for a while: the fear, the pity, and the horror in people's eyes. In fact, I'd meet someone who'd give me a limp handshake and I'd immediately see all the other faces with pity and horror in their eyes.

I didn't want to hang onto this horror and pain anymore. I didn't want to think of it every day of my life. So I stopped. Every time I went outside, and every time I saw that look in people's eyes, I chose to ignore it and walk with confidence. These days, I don't see those same reactions, maybe in part because others see the confidence in me.

A few years ago, I began speaking in schools. It all began with an invite from a teacher friend of mine to speak to his class. Then a teacher from another school heard about my talk and invited me to talk to her class. From there, a few invites a year came from elementary schools, junior high, and high schools. Today I'm invited once a year by the local university to speak to occupational therapy students.

At the beginning, I was a nervous wreck before each speaking engagement, but once I got going I found myself relaxed and free of anxiety. I gave students the opportunity to ask questions after each talk. The most common questions had to do with what happened to the teens who threw the firecrackers that night.

Children in the lower grades always asked the best questions. Once the ice was broken, hands would shoot up all over the classroom: "What can you do?"

I would explain that I could do anything I needed to. I could do anything they could do.

"Why does your nose look that way?"

"Good question. It looks a little crooked, doesn't it? I'm not really sure why."

As far as I was concerned, answering the questions was always the highlight of the talk.

Belief in God played a big role in my home, and for years it was more my parents' belief that I carried around.

It wasn't so much that I didn't believe in God but that he didn't often feel real to me.

There were a few times in my life when God *did* seem absolutely real, and remained real from then on. The first such time was when I hurt my back playing soccer. The pain plagued me for years. My chiropractor said that only time could cure it. I'd be fine for a while, but then something would aggravate my lower back and I'd be in intense pain for weeks.

One day, while helping my mom, I picked up a thirty-pound bag improperly and re-pulled that muscle. It just happened that the church I was going to had started a week of prayer. Every evening for an hour, a few folks showed up. I was in such obvious pain that each night they prayed for my back, but nothing happened.

On the last evening of the week, I was again prayed for. This time I felt the pain disappear as people prayed for me. It just went away and I never felt pain there again. I always attributed that to God's great love for me.

The latest time God seemed real to me was in the writing of this book. He gave me a peace such as I've never experienced to walk away from my day job in 2006 and write full-time with only my meager savings to live off. Once I left my job, I began to get ideas for writing several more books. I lived off less per month than I did while working, but I was suddenly somehow able to afford things I couldn't before.

*   *   *

When I was out in public, anger would rise up when I saw people staring at me. I had a choice to make. Would I push into anger? Would I use the anger to get me through those hard times? Or would I walk away? If I pushed into anger, I would become an angry boy, and from there grow into an angry man. Instead I chose to just walk away.

I had many such crossroads in my life, crossroads where I would choose to go either left or right. One other such choice was this: should I choose to be excited for others when they do well, or not? I chose yes. It is amazing to me how happy I could then feel when someone accomplished something big. Choosing this route made life so much more pleasant and exciting.

Another was whether to take offense or not take offense. I found that when offenses got right in my face, I could refuse to take them and they'd disappear harmlessly. I learned from this that being offended or not being offended is a choice.

I made the choice not to let people's stares and comments bother me. After that, I found that I no longer noticed it. When I was with friends, they would sometimes mention it, and I would realize that it no longer bothered me.

Once I started a job, I found myself confronted with a new choice. Would I be a conscientious worker or not? I chose to be. I realized after I'd worked at it for awhile that a conscientious worker works just as hard when the boss is away as when the boss is around.

At one point in my life, I started noticing different blocks in my life. I had the choice to work out a few of these problems in my life or not. I decided to go for it and set out to find a good counselor. It was rather a circuitous route towards recovery, and not all of it was enjoyable.

One day, I noticed that small things were making me see red. It was then that I realized I had a lot of anger in me. The very next day, I was invited over to a friend's house for a visit with a few others. When I arrived, she was just into a tale about a course she'd taken where she learned to deal with her anger. When I asked her about it, she gave me all the information.

"Just phone this number," she said, handing me a piece of paper. "Tell whoever answers that you want to sign up for the twelve-week course."

I called the very next day and was told the class was full but that the teacher always reserved a few seats. He'd give me a call, and if he felt I really needed to attend the course he'd put me in the class.

Two days later, I got a call from the office and was informed that I was in the class. A friend of mine had signed up as well, so we carpooled together; it was about an hour's drive away.

We arrived excited for our first class only to find out it wasn't the course we thought it was. Turned out we had accidently signed up for a twelve-week counseling course, and when I found that out I was hopping mad!

I stayed for the course, though, and through it saw different areas in myself that I could now identify as some of the major road blocks in my life.

At the end of the twelve weeks, the teacher informed us that he did one-on-one counseling but only took new clients if they had taken one of his courses. So now I qualified!

I quickly made an appointment and was much happier about having ended up in the wrong course.

One of the blocks in my life was a problem with authority. It stemmed from my time in the hospital, particularly the run-ins I had with a couple of nurses: the one who ripped me away from the railing when saying my long, drawn-out farewell to my mom, and the nurse who promised to soak the dressing off my leg and then ripped it right off. I chose to forgive those two and the problem with authority subsided. It was an amazing feeling to let this pain and resentment fall away.

I started liking myself better after I got rid of these blocks in my life. Resolving these problems didn't fill me with pride, but I went from one side of the spectrum to the other—from not really caring who I was or how I looked, to seeing that yes, I was disfigured, but I liked who I was.

The anger was now gone as well. Things went so much smoother when I wasn't getting upset over life. I like what God had done in my life.

I never met the boys who started the fire, but to my knowledge no charges were brought against them. They were under the age of sixteen at the time and the fire was not intentional. I don't feel anything against them. I don't hold them responsible for anything that I had to go through: for all the times people treated me as inferior or for those who refused to give me jobs because of my appearance, for the startled gasps and screams I received from people when I was out in public.

No, those boys were not responsible for how people treated me afterwards. Were I to meet them today, I would want them to know that I do not hold anything against them, though their actions, meant as a practical joke, did start my life on this altered path.

I would say, "I understand that it was a practical joke, and I know you didn't even realize what it was you had done until later. Regardless of that, it changed my life. It shows how wrong a practical joke can go. I've struggled through many things in my life, and yet I like the person I've become. For your part in this, I tell you that I don't hold anything against you. I don't see the fire as planned and intentional. I could blame you for the hardness of my life, but I choose not to. I forgive you and I hope you can put this all behind you now."

CHAPTER 23

PURE DETERMINATION

Dave

My mom didn't tell me this until I was an adult, but the doctors declared that I would always be totally handicapped with my hands. This would have been too harsh to tell me as a child.

The following is the medical report written by my plastic surgeon a year and a half after the fire:

December 20, 1973

Dear Sirs,

RE: Hammer, Keir
Hammer, Dave

As you must realize the charts on both these boys are very, very extensive and involve numerous hospi-

tal admissions and hospital procedures. I will try and arrange all this into a reasonable order, attempting to be concise, however not leaving out any signifying details. Both these patients have been under Dr. Maxwell's care and Dr. Timmons's care. It was in early July that I became involved with both. I will however also summarize Dr. Timmons's material as I have his records. I will deal with Keir Hammer first.

On May 22, 1972, this boy was burned in a tent fire in St. Albert. He was initially taken to the Sturgeon General Hospital where he was quickly transferred to the Royal Alexandra Hospital. It was estimated that body burns were between 30% and 40% total body surface and most of these were third degree burns. The principle areas involved were the entire face, both arms including hands and almost the entire dorsal except for the right lateral chest. There were very few burns below the waist. These were small in area. He was resuscitated in the ICU, transferred to the ward at a suitable time. Because of the extensive burns a large amount of management was involved in the case. On June 14, he was first taken to the Operating Room, at that time skin grafts were applied to arms, neck and face.

As for Dave Hammer, he was burned on the same day as his brother. His burns and condition of admission were much more extensive than his older brother's. Burns involved approximately 60% of his total body surface, all the areas above the waist were third degree burned. The only area on his upper body that did not have third degree burn was a small area on the *back of his neck. It was obvious at the time of admission (photographs were taken) that he would lose all the ends of his fingers and both thumbs. He did undergo a cardiac arrest the night of admission and was resuscitated. It was at this time that a tracheostomy was being performed by Dr. Maxwell. He was an extremely ill little boy for several months following admission. He spent a long time in the ICU before being transferred to a ward. On the ward he was still a considerable amount of work. From June 8, until July 12, he was taken to the Operating Room on six occasions by Dr. Timmons. Surgery consisted of debridement of burns, dressing changes, and beginnings of skin grafts to arms, face and chest. I first began managing this boy in the middle of July, 1972. Since then he has had an additional twenty-four trips to the Operating Room, one of these was by Dr. Timmons and the remainder by myself. Surgery dates are July 16, July 20, July 25, July 31, August 4, August 10, August 18, August 23, August 30, September 6, September 16, September 21, October 2, October 13, and October 25, all consisted of debridements of burns, dressing changes, and multiple skin grafts to the burned areas. Also during this course all his fingers were amputated because of dry gangrene due to the burns. He was a continual management problem throughout. During the later part of this arrangements were made for him to attend the Glenrose Hospital. He was initially managed there as an In-patient also. Since then he has returned to the Royal Alexandra Hospital on five occasions to be admitted. There has been nine surgi-*

cal procedures performed, for reconstruction. Surgery
has been further grafting to his scalp, reconstruction
of semi-functional hands, and release of scar contractures in both axxilla, his neck and his face. At present he is still attending the Glenrose School for the
Handicapped, is living at home now, and is still under
my care.

As to his present status, he is a very badly scarred
and deformed boy for life. He will never grow any
hair on his scalp as it is entire skin grafts. His face
is permanently scarred. He will probably have problems with exposure of his eyes for many years. We
anticipate further reconstruction in this area. His
face is very badly scarred. His neck is equally as bad
as he has scar contracture in both axillae. His arms
are total skin grafts. He has stubs of fingers present on both hands. At present neither hand is very
functional, they certainly do not look normal. Much
reconstruction is needed here. The remainder of his entire body is totally scarred from skin grafting or donor
areas. These will remain so for the rest of his life.

Keir Hammer I believe is finished with any reconstruction of a surgical nature. Perhaps some minor
revisions may be performed around his mouth. It will
be at least one to two years before a decision will be
made on this.

As for Dave Hammer, multiple procedures will
still have to be done. He is booked for more reconstruction surgery early in the New Year. It is a constant battle with him, releasing scar contractures and
skin grafting. He has no good available skin left and

we are using used donor areas for skin grafting. This produces less than ideal results and many procedures often have to be repeated. There is work needed on his lower lids as he cannot close his eyes, and is continually getting an exposure keratitis. His scalp is still not completely healed. When this is healed a suitable wig will be obtained which will improve him somewhat. Scars in his neck will again have to be released at a later date. The tight burn scars on his face have produced some deformity of his jaws, and in time he will have dental problems also. More scar contractures will be released in both axillae in time. His biggest problem at present is his hands. Many operative procedures and many episodes of skin grafting will have to be performed before the best functional result for him can be obtained. Nevertheless the end result on his hands will be poor and he always will be totally handicapped with these.

I hope the above information is suitable for you. If not I will be certainly happy to furnish more. As you must realize the charts on both these boys are very extensive and the above is only a summary of the total involvement.

If I can be of any further assistance please don't hesitate to call on me.

Yours sincerely,
Dr. Strazinsky M.D.

Not wanting to crush my spirits, my mom didn't say a word about this letter until I was an adult. She watched me struggle to do simple things, then struggle to do everything. She always thought, years later, that the doctors would never believe all that I learned to do.

When I was born, the doctor who delivered me said to my parents, "Look at those hands. He's going to be a basketball player!" But my hands didn't grow much after the fire and my fingers were mere stubs. Therefore, when I became full grown, they were still quite small. My hands might have been big at birth, but because of the fire the skin was too tight to allow any growth.

My mom watched me struggle through everything. First I needed to be fed, and then I tried hard to feed myself with straps. This was difficult, because although I could handle the spoon strapped to my hand, I wasn't able to get much food into my mouth. The length of the spoon was throwing me off and it was hard to balance the spoon in the strap. With it, though, I was able to feed myself better.

Slowly, with grit and determination, my mom watched me master the act of feeding myself. Then one day, at the age of six, I decided to start living without the help of straps. This became easier as I built up strength in my hands, which hadn't been used much in over a year.

Looking back, my mom still remembers me sitting in my hospital bed, day after day, with not much to do aside from looking at the hospital ward as my domain to conquer. Once I saw things from this perspective, nothing held me back.

Soon I was feeding myself quite easily without the straps, and once I was rid of them I didn't seem to need any special tools at all.

Originally, the occupational therapy department gave me an all-Velcro wardrobe to help me dress myself. Once I mastered Velcro, I asked for shirts with big buttons. It took me a little while, but eventually I perfected doing those buttons up. From there, I learned to work small buttons, zippers, snaps, and hooks. I became adept at doing up zippers on pants and jackets.

My older brother Keir told me that he was always amazed at how quick I became at doing up buttons. He has all his fingers and says he doesn't find them as easy as I seem to.

Next, I switched to learning to tie my shoes. I wanted to be totally independent and wear shoes with laces. It took me awhile, but finally I could do it. I wasn't quick, but at least I could do it. My mom recalls that I was so excited once I could tie my own shoes that I had a big grin on my face.

She was amazed that I didn't become frustrated learning to do new things. She tells me I had a patience and persistence that was awe-inspiring. She goes on to recount that she doesn't remember ever thinking of anything specific that I would not be able to do. I would look up at the steep incline of each new mountain, then begin to climb, and eventually succeed.

Except for a few years of burying my nose in books and struggling with self-pity, I didn't isolate myself. I marched right out there and faced the world with a positive attitude.

So many people have told me how amazed they are not only at how much I can do, but at how well I can do it. When I meet someone for the first time, based upon my appearance and the condition of my hands, they don't think I can do much. When they realize I can do as much as anyone, they start to look at me in a different light.

A child once asked, "Can you write?"

"Yes," the person with me replied. "Probably even better than you can."

In fact, once people get to know me, they start thinking, like me, that I am no different than anyone else. I am so grateful for the people who treat me the way *they* like to be treated, right from the start.

My good friends saw me simply for me. This was especially apparent when they learned that my driver training fees were covered.

When I told the story years later, my friends Don and Louise looked intrigued.

"How much did it cost?" Don asked when I'd finished.

"It was free."

Don looked a little skeptical. "Free?"

"Yes, because I'm handicapped."

"You are not handicapped!" Louise said quickly. Her retort practically exploded from her mouth.

In contrast, many people still watch me do things and wonder how I do them, because I am so different. My mom has a clear memory of wondering how I was going to manage learning to ride a bike. She recalls my tenacious "never give up" attitude. When I outgrew my first bike, Mom bought me a bigger one. As she watched me, she'd wonder, *How on earth does he hang on to those handlebars?*

Years later, I was mountain-biking with Russ, my friend from high school. We often rode together and that day we rode over the bumpiest, roughest trail yet. During the ride, Russ pulled alongside me because he had to ask, "How are you able to hang on to the handlebars?"

"By pure determination," I told him.

That's how I did everything—by pure determination!

I did more than my parents could have ever imagined. As my mom watched me accomplishing things she never thought I'd try, she concluded that just because something can't be imagined does not mean it isn't possible.

I played basketball and had an awesome shot. I wasn't bad at dribbling, either, at least not in the early years. As the scar tissue tightened up on my hands, pulling my left thumb down towards my palm, dribbling became more difficult. I was fine dribbling on my own, but if I had to make quick or fancy moves, my dexterity failed me.

In order to write, I originally had to press my two palms together with a pen between them. It looked awkward, yet I had neat penmanship. My mom was amazed at *how* I did things, not so much that I could do them. My challenges greatly stimulated my creativity, and I accomplished feats that might otherwise have been impossible.

At my call center job, I decided to teach myself to write with only one hand. This facilitated my writing in that I was then able to hold a piece of paper in place while I wrote.

When I started this process, I wrote with my left hand. At first my writing was a bit crude, but not too bad. But after a few months of sticking to it, my penmanship was just as neat as ever. Today I sometimes revert back to the two-handed method if I'm doing a lot of writing because it saves me from getting a hand cramp.

In the early years, I struggled to do things most people take for granted, yet later I targeted the activities people told me I wouldn't be able to do. These accomplishments have given me strong confidence in life.

I left home when I was sixteen, young for anyone but particularly for someone who'd been through so much trauma. Mom had left home at age seventeen to attend college. She boarded a train, with only a trunk and suitcase, destined for Macalester College in St Paul, Minnesota. That's all she knew. And yet she couldn't imagine me going away at age sixteen, headed to a strange new place where I had no idea how I'd be received. She was proud of my bravery, particularly in light of the psychologist's words: "Dave will be totally dependent on you for the next fifty to seventy years."

Barely eleven years after the Glenrose psychologist spoke those words, I packed up and moved away from home to attend high school three hours away.

Over the years, my mom watched me learn to do all the things that boys learn to do and, as I grew into a man, learned to do the things that came with that, too, like driving a car and going to work everyday. The characteristic she has noticed most is that I've always lived as if I'm unaware of my handicap; I've always thought of myself as the same as any other person in the world.

*   *   *

As I wrote this book, I found people telling me what they found amazing about me. I didn't ask them; they simply volunteered it. I find it hard to see those things in myself, because to me I'm normal. It doesn't seem amazing to me to be able to do everything the same as anyone else.

One of my co-workers told me, "After all you've been through, it's so amazing how normal you are."

A classmate from college reflected, "One of my clearest memories of you is your positive attitude toward everything. I'll never forget the time our class was expected to sing a children's song and perform the actions, an activity to which I failed to see the point. However, in the midst of my disgust, you leaned over towards me and whispered, 'Get into it.' Not only was your cheerful heart good medicine, but the memory has brought me many smiles and cheer over the years. One of the things that stands out the most about your positive attitude and sense of humor is that it didn't stem from a flippant, goofy approach to life from someone who had it all easy. In spite of your pain and suffering, more than most of us can imagine, you obviously made the remarkable choice to honor God with a good attitude. Of the countless people your positive spirit has blessed and taught, I am grateful to be one of them."

A good friend said, "You have so many reasons to be angry, and yet you choose not to be."

Another classmate from college recently informed me, "Of all the people I know, you're one of the few who is secure with who you are. And that says a lot, because everyone else I know has issues they can hide or try to control. Yours stares you in the face every morning."

*   *   *

Now that you've read my story and learned of all the obstacles I've had to overcome, I want to encourage you that there is no trial *you* can't overcome. I'm not superhuman, I've just learned to never give up on myself, to never stop trying. I hope you do, too.

EPILOGUE

I passed through the flames into a totally new life. It began as a harsher, harder life, but it didn't stay that way. I changed a lot over the years; I became less competitive, got rid of my anger, began using my humor again, learning to balance it with my serious side, and learned to enjoy life. I went from being one girl's hero (trying to ignore the reality of my altered appearance) to finally seeing myself honestly. Once I faced who I really was, I was able to truly start liking myself. That's when freedom flowed, and I grasped the truth that being different in some ways didn't have to isolate me from this world in any way.

I have come to grips with my pain and my appearance. I love life more and more and my life became easier and more pleasant as I changed within. I like who I've become.

My life isn't hard now. It isn't easy, either. Things don't just fall into my lap, at least not so far. But it's not a hard life, because I choose to focus on the positive.

I also don't live life with a sour expression. Why should I? I enjoy life, and I don't live as if someone owes me a favor. Sometimes people can be rude, but for the most part I understand that people are curious when they see me for the first time, and I choose daily not to take offense at that. I now walk confidently in public. I live on my own and buy groceries and clothes. I go out for coffee, to the movies, to the mall, and to eat, and I feel like I belong there. I don't even seem to get negative reactions like I used to, or perhaps I just don't notice them as much now.

I have a wonderful, supportive family. Good friends, too...friends who support me when I take bold steps and do things that they don't always identify with, such as leaving my job to be a writer. I'm so glad I listened to God's leading voice, as I feel more like "me" than I ever did working a forty-hour week. I'm thankful for the support around me as I push myself hard towards my goals.

When it comes to pursuing my dreams, I see myself as I see others: a person with a future and goals to pursue. I make decisions without my handicap in the forefront. I could have passed on trying many things, yet to me it is much better to try. You never know what might be possible!

My outlook on life hasn't been that I *can't* do anything (I wouldn't have tried anything with that attitude), and it hasn't been that I *can* do everything (or I would have faced endless disappointment), but that I would *try* everything to see what I can do.

Don't give up on the things in your heart. It will limit your life. I hope my story can be an inspiration to you. When you stop letting life beat you up and follow your heart passionately and confidently, it's possible to rise above the impossible and lead a happy and fulfilling life. Trust me. You'll be surprised what you discover.

APPENDIX

RCMP confirm fireworks caused fatal tent fire

RCMP confirmed today that youths throwing firecrackers caused a tent fire which killed two St. Albert girls Sunday.

A spokesman said RCMP took statements from three juveniles in connection with the incident, but no charges would be laid unless the attorney-general's department so directed.

Dianne Rosenburg, 10, of 69 Garden Cres., and Kimberley Hammer, 9, of 71 Garden Cres., died after fire swept through a tent in which they were sleeping in the back yard of the Hammer residence.

Three other children were injured in the fire. Bruce Hammer, 5, and Keir Hammer, 7, are both still in serious c o n d i t i o n in hospital, while the condition of Karen Bergman, 10, of 70 Garden Cres., has improved from poor to satisfactory.

Journal, Wed, May 24, 1972

Coroner's Report

CANADA
Province of Alberta }
To Wit:

An Inquisition taken for our Sovereign Lady the Queen at the house of ....Town Hall........
__Council Chambers_____ in the _____TOWN_____ of __ST. ALBERT__
  (Thursday)
on the (1:30 P.M.) _29th_ day of ____JUNE_____ 19 72 (and by adjournment on the
_____ day of _____ 19 ____), before _____
__DR. MAX M. CANTOR_____ one of the Coroners of our said Lady the Queen for the Pro-
                        Kimberly HANNER and
vince of Alberta, on view of the body of ___Diane Jane ROSENBERG_____ , then and there
lying dead, the undersigned _____

good and lawful men, being duly sworn, and charged to inquire for our said Lady the Queen, when,
                                    Kimberly HANNER and
where, how and by what means the said __Diane Jane ROSENBERG__   9
                                                                     10
_____ ST. ALBERT _____ came to _____their_____ death, do upon their oath say: (Age)
        (Residence)

Time: ___About 2:30 A.M. May 21st 1972_____

Place: __In a tent at the rear of #70 Garden Crescent, St. Albert, Alberta._____

Cause: __Acute asphyxia by anoxia and incineration_____

Circumstances: __The two deceased were sleeping in a canvas tent with three other__
__children when the tent was ignited by the sparks or smouldering remains of two__
__or three firecrackers thrown into the area of the tent entrance by one of three__
__juveniles acting together.__

Opinion and Recommendations: _1) Both deceased died from accidental burns as noted__
__in a 12 year old canvas tent which was untreated to make it fire resistant, and__
__that the tent occupants were in no way responsible for the fire.__
__2) The sale of firecrackers and similar fireworks should be prohibited to any__
__person regardless of age, ____ __ _____ _____/__
__3) That firecrackers and other fireworks should be prohibited from sale through__
__ordinary outlets such as retail stores, etc.__
__4) That firecrackers and other fireworks should be sold only through specified__
__sources and then only to a person responsible for their use at public exhibitions__
__or fairs to be used only under proper fire safety supervision having first obtained__
__a permit for such use from the local fire commissioner.__
IN WITNESS WHEREOF, the Coroner has hereunto set his hand and the Jury have hereto
set their hands this _____29th_____ day of _____June_____ 19 72.

_____ (Foreman)

_____ Juror

_____ Juror   CERTIFIED TRUE COPY

_____ Juror   _____
                                        B. D. Sturrock (Coroner)
_____ Juror

_____ Juror

                                        _____
                                        A Coroner in and for the Province of Alberta.

5) That materials used in construction of sleeping
bags and tents be required to meet at
least minimum fire resistant standards.

A.G. 304
V. 1211

AUTHOR'S NOTE

These events are as accurate as possible according to the information gathered. I wrote the first several chapters from several people's point of view, doing my best to put myself in their shoes. My mom provided some letters written by my grandma and some of her sisters in the months following the fire. The purpose of those letters was to keep the family informed, and they became very instrumental in recreating what took place in the hospital during my initial recovery period, when I was unconscious.

I chose to write Chapter Nine in the third-person, from the point of view of multiple characters. Except for my decision to write one of the boys as having led the others, the details of how the fire started are based on information gathered from legal documents I had access to.

Before 1980, few serious burn victims survived their accidents. Medical advances have made it possible, even for a person with over 90% of their body burned, to survive. Canadian Burn Foundation continues to work with burn survivors and their families to enable them to live life as best they can under their challenging circumstances. (www.canadianburnfoundation.org)

ABOUT THE AUTHOR

Dave Hammer (pronounced haw-mer) is a graduate of Taylor University College in Edmonton, Alberta, Canada. He left his day job in 2006 to pursue writing full-time. He currently lives in Western Canada.

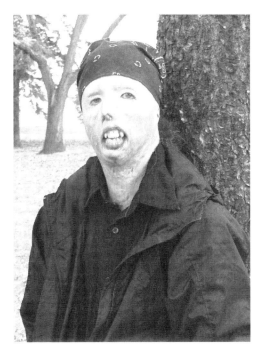

Photo by Wayne Teskey